OECD Reviews of Health Systems: Lithuania 2018

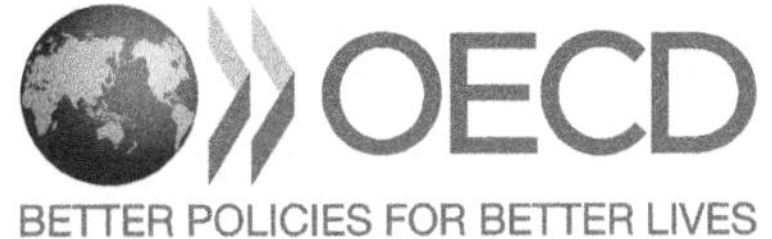

Please cite this publication as:
OECD (2018), *OECD Reviews of Health Systems: Lithuania 2018*, OECD Publishing, Paris
http://dx.doi.org/10.1787/9789264300873-en

ISBN 978-92-64-30086-6 (print)
ISBN 978-92-64-30087-3 (PDF)

Series: OECD Reviews of Health Systems
ISSN 1990-1429 (print)
ISSN 1990-1410 (online)

Photo credits: Cover © Rimantas Zagrebajev, Ministry of Health, Lithuania.

Corrigenda to OECD publications may be found on line at: *www.oecd.org/about/publishing/corrigenda.htm*.

Foreword

Lithuania has made remarkable progress in reshaping its health system since the 1990s. The institutional and legal framework for providing health services is solid and well-functioning. An important component is the social health insurance system, partly funded by general budget resources to cover the non-active population, which has proven resilient in the face of the financial crisis and provides broadly adequate and equitable access to health services. Despite spending only 6.5% of GDP on health, admission rates and physician visits are well above OECD averages and unmet needs are just below the OECD average.

Lithuania has also developed a primary care system with many features which deserve to be recognised as examples for other OECD countries, including expanded nurses' practice and primary care centres with an effective gatekeeping role. Although there is still excess hospital capacity, the reform agenda for the hospital sector, involving clustering and concentration of services into larger units to raise the quality and efficiency of delivery is promising. The same is true for recent efforts to strengthen public health through policies to curb risk factors, in particular the harmful and exceptionally high alcohol consumption.

Nevertheless, Lithuania needs to decisively address a number of challenges. Life expectancy is rising slowly, but remains almost six years below the OECD average, with a large gender gap. Data on the health status of the population show that if more effective public health and medical interventions were in place, fewer people would die prematurely in Lithuania. In other words, the mix and quality of interventions delivered must improve.

Greater use of performance data to increase accountability would support these objectives. Decisive implementation of health reforms needs to be accompanied by systematic evaluations to understand how to achieve better results quickly. Deepening the use and analysis of the already rich data available in the country and further efforts to foster a culture of transparency of results would help in holding stakeholders accountable for performance, and help Lithuania building further on its already significant achievements.

This review was prepared by the OECD Secretariat to support the OECD Health Committee's evaluation of Lithuania's health system, undertaken as part of the process for Lithuania's accession to the OECD (see Roadmap for the Accession of Lithuania to the OECD [C(2015)92/FINAL]). In accordance with paragraph 14 of the Roadmap, the Health Committee agreed to declassify the review and publish it in order to allow a wider audience to become acquainted with the issues raised in the review. Publication of this document and the analysis and recommendations contained therein, does not prejudge in any way the results of the ongoing review of Lithuania as part of its process of accession to the OECD.

Acknowledgements

This Health system review was written, managed and co-ordinated by Agnès Couffinhal. The other authors of the report are Jens Wilkens and Karolina Socha-Dietrich. The authors wish to thank Mark Pearson, Francesca Colombo and Stefano Scarpetta from the OECD Directorate of Employment, Labour and Social affairs for their detailed comments and suggestions as well as Ruth Lopert and Kate Cornford for their insights and review. Thanks also to Duniya Dedeyn and Lucy Hulett for editing support.

The OECD Secretariat would like to thank the Lithuanian authorities for their outstanding support throughout the process of this review. The process had the full support of the Ministry's leadership, first Vice-Ministers Valentin Gavrilov and Jūratė Sabalienė and subsequently Minister Aurelijus Veryga. All the staff at the International Cooperation Division, most notably, Radvilė Jakaitienė deserve special thanks for their contributions to organising the initial fact-finding mission in November 2016 and their commitment to ensuring the authors liaise with counterparts in the Lithuanian health system throughout the project. The OECD Secretariat is also grateful to all the people who have been interviewed, provided data, and responded to detailed questions very responsively. Invaluable information and thorough explanations of the Lithuanian health system have been provided by many staff in the Ministry's Healthcare Resources and Innovation Management Department, the Pharmacy Department, the Health Economics Department, the Personal Healthcare Department, the Public Healthcare Department, the Drug, Tobacco and Alcohol Control Department, and the Legal Department. Numerous representatives from the National Health Insurance Fund, the State Medicines Control Agency, the Institute of Hygiene, and the State Health Care Accreditation Agency have contributed greatly with information and insights. Valuable information has also been provided by staff from the Ministry of Finance, the Ministry of Foreign Affairs, and the Office of the Prime Minister. The review has benefitted from comments of Lithuanian authorities who reviewed earlier drafts.

During the initial mission the review team also greatly benefitted from fruitful meetings with the health and social municipality administrations of Druskininkai, as well as representatives of the local hospital, PHC Centre and Public Health Bureau. Furthermore, very informative interviews were conducted with key organisations providing important insights, including the Lithuanian Nurses' Organization, the Lithuanian General Practitioner's Society, the Vilnius University Hospital, the Lithuanian Hospital Managers Association, the Lithuanian Hospital Association, the Medicines Manufacturer's Association, the local American Working Group, the Innovative Pharmaceutical Industry association, the Help of Cancer Patients Association, and the Order of Malta Relief Organization.

Table of contents

Tables

Figures

Acronyms and abbreviations

ALOS	Average Length of Stay
AMR	Antimicrobial Resistance
ECDC	European Centre for Disease Prevention and Control
EHIS	European Health Interview Survey
EU-NMS	European Union new member states
GDP	Gross domestic product
HTA	Health technology assessment
INN	International Non-proprietary Name
MHC	Mental healthcare centers
MOH	Ministry of Health
NHIF	National Health Insurance Fund
OECD	Organisation for Economic Co-operation and Development
OOP	Out-of-pocket payments
PHC	Primary Health Care
SHCAA	State Health Care Accreditation Agency
WHO	World Health Organization

In figures, "OECD" refers to the unweighted average of OECD countries for which data are available.

Executive summary

Since the re-establishment of the country's independence, Lithuania's health system has been profoundly reorganised. In the early 1990s, the system was exclusively public, centrally planned, financially integrated and hospital-centric. Ownership has since been diversified, reforms have sought to rebalance service delivery by developing primary health care and restructuring the hospital system, modernising payment systems, and introducing modern regulations.

Although spending is low, the system provides broadly adequate and equitable access to care. At 6.5% of GDP, Lithuania's health spending remains below that of countries with a similar income per capita. In general, the laws and regulations in the Lithuanian health sector have proven effective in maintaining public health budgets within planned parameters. Projections indicate that spending is not expected to increase as quickly as in many other fast-ageing economies.

A well-run health insurance fund provides coverage to virtually the entire population. It contracts with autonomous providers, including an emerging private sector. The state guarantees and funds access to coverage for the economically inactive. This served as a powerful counter-cyclical financing mechanism when the 2008 global financial crisis hit.

Even if out-of-pocket payments represent nearly a third of health spending in Lithuania, the system broadly ensures access to care.

- Admission rates and physician visits are well above OECD averages, unmet needs are just below the OECD average and differences across socio-economic groups are not stark.
- Waiting lists exist for some specialised services but rationing is not a common feature of the system.
- Ambulatory drugs are extensively funded through out-of-pocket payments and there are indications patients do not systematically use the cheapest medicines available. In 2014, only 2% of the population reported that they had not followed a prescription because of the cost.
- In 2016, one in 4 of patients still declare paying informally for care, 10 percentage points less than four years before but among the highest proportions in the EU.
- A more detailed diagnostic on possible barriers to access would require better data on waiting times and out-of-pocket payments for medicines.

The main challenge to the health system is that health outcomes still place Lithuania among the lowest ranked in the OECD.

- Life expectancy at birth is nearly six years below the OECD average (close to the levels in Mexico and Latvia), and characterised by a larger gender gap than in any OECD country.

- Chronic conditions account for the majority of deaths, and excess mortality due to cardio-vascular diseases and suicide are more than double the OECD average.
- While the burden of disease is similar to countries in the region, some of them have achieved more rapid progress (e.g. Estonia, the Slovak Republic).

Many structural elements and policies are already in place in Lithuania to address these challenges, but the efficiency of spending and quality of service delivered in primary care, hospital care, and public health must improve rapidly.

Primary health care (PHC) is well developed and reflects best OECD practices.

- PHC physicians work in teams with nurses – whose role is expanding – and are expected to provide care after hours.
- Patients have to register with a gatekeeping PHC provider, and information is available on individual facilities' performance to guide their choice of provider.
- PHC providers receive a capitation payment combined with fees incentivising the delivery of preventive services, as well as a pay-for-performance element.

PHC's capacity to manage patients care is improving, as shown by the decreasing proportion of patients hospitalised for some of the conditions which should, on the whole, be managed by PHC providers, such as asthma and congestive heart failure. However, absolute levels of hospitalisations remain high and the coverage of some preventive services, in particular cancer screening, is low. Care co-ordination also needs strengthening.

The health system remains too hospital-centric. Despite restructuring, Lithuania is still one of the countries with the highest number of beds (and hospitalisations) per capita in the OECD, and the bed occupancy ratio is below the OECD average in 85% of hospitals. Further, many facilities still perform very few surgeries and deliveries, which is inefficient but also carries a risk for patients, as facilities delivering lower volume tend to have worse outcomes of care.

Hospital contracting seeks to incentivise efficiency. In particular, diagnosis-related prices per case encourage the efficient use of resources within hospitals. Contracts are based on slowly decreasing volume caps to encourage a shift away from inpatient care, but day-case volumes are not capped to encourage this form of service delivery.

Two recent initiatives hold the potential to improve both quality and efficiency in hospitals. First, contracting for surgery and maternity is now limited to hospitals providing more than a minimum volume of services. Second, standardised pathways have been introduced for stroke and some myocardial infarctions, and specialised centres offer previously under-developed services. Further consolidation of the hospital network requires more active planning of service delivery across municipalities and reducing the influence of local governments in decision-making.

Finally, a sustainable reduction in the burden of disease requires additional investment in public health. Curbing unhealthy behaviours, such as harmful drinking and smoking, particularly among men, is necessary to close the gap with high performing OECD countries. The importance of public health is recognised among decision-makers, but more systematic efforts are required. Health features as a prominent inter-sectoral priority across Lithuania's strategic planning documents, and the health strategy emphasises the importance of tackling health determinants and reducing inequalities. At the same time, stakeholders are not effectively held accountable for progress on public health, and actual initiatives tend to be small-scale, seldom evaluated and short-lived.

Across the sector, further investments will be needed to accelerate progress on outcomes. These will need to be systematically directed towards high-impact interventions. There is remarkable consensus among stakeholders in Lithuania behind priorities which are aligned with the burden of disease and reforms which are conducive to achieving these objectives, but more decisive and better sustained efforts are needed.

Priority areas to improve health outcomes include:

- Further pursue and deepen efforts to rationalise the use of hospital resources and rebalance service delivery, with greater emphasis on care co-ordination and mental health at PHC level;
- Invest effectively in public health to tackle risk factors, notably harmful alcohol consumption;
- Develop a quality assurance culture to better measure results and hold stakeholders more explicitly accountable for improving them;
- Scale up the system's capacity to evaluate the impact of policies and understand the reasons for their success or lack thereof.

Assessment and recommendations

The organisation of the health system of Lithuania is modern and characterised by institutional stability. The country has been steadily pursuing policies designed to better tackle the burden of chronic diseases, including for instance the development of primary care. Remarkably, and despite the fact that Lithuania spends little on health, the population benefits from quasi-universal coverage and key metrics suggest access to care is broadly adequate.

The main challenge Lithuania continues to face however is that the health of the population is not improving as fast as it has in comparable countries and many outcome indicators place it among the poor performers of the OECD. There is scope to improve the efficiency of resources currently allocated to the sector as well as the quality and outcomes of care. Additional investments in health are probably also warranted and would not necessarily undermine system's sustainability but they need to be systematically geared towards addressing the challenges identified.

In all spheres of health policy, a more decisive implementation of reforms needs to be accompanied with systematic evaluations to understand what may or may not work, why and what course-adjustments might be required to achieve better results faster.

This opening chapter summarises the in-depth assessment carried out in the context of Lithuania's accession review and formulates key recommendations to improve the performance of the health system in the key dimensions of sustainability, access, efficiency and quality.

Lithuania's health system has modernised but health outcomes continue to be poor

Lithuania's economy is dynamic but faces some socio-demographic challenges

After the collapse of the central planning system in 1991, Lithuania experienced a difficult but fast transition towards a market economy. Economic growth was sustained in the transition phase above that of many OECD countries. Nevertheless, the economy has been vulnerable to external shocks and the impact of the global financial crisis of 2008 was severe, with a drop in GDP of nearly 15% and unemployment surging up to 18% in 2009. Since 2011, economic growth has once again been of the highest among European as well as OECD countries.

Despite impressive progress, Lithuania still faces serious socio-economic challenges. The share of the population at risk of poverty is the third highest among European countries. The poverty is also deep-rooted as the income of the poor is on average 23% below the poverty line. Lithuania is also one of the fastest-ageing countries in the EU. Indeed, the working-age population is projected to shrink by nearly half between 2014 and 2050 a trend largely driven by relatively high mortality and very strong emigration among adults aged 25-64 years.

The health system is well-designed and institutionally stable

Along with economic progress, Lithuania has achieved a profound transformation of its health system in the decades following independence. When it declared independence in the early 1990s, Lithuania's health system was typical of the Soviet era: an exclusively public, centrally-planned, financially integrated, hospital-centric service delivery system provided curative services to the entire population. In the following decade, increasing autonomy was granted to state hospitals, and municipal management and ownership was introduced for out-patient services and local hospitals. The compulsory health insurance legislation in 1996 was a milestone in moving towards a contractual model with a third-party payer and relatively autonomous providers.

The organisation and governance of the system today are typical of many European countries, and have been remarkably stable in the past 20 years. The Ministry of Health (MoH) and the National Health Insurance Fund (NHIF) are the main central institutions, with local administrations playing an important role in service delivery. The MoH supported by a handful of specialised agencies formulates health policy and regulations. Insurance coverage is provided to the population by the NHIF. In order to obtain coverage, the active population must contribute to the NHIF. The economically inactive, including children and students, pensioners and the unemployed, constituting 54% of the population in 2016, are automatically covered. The NHIF purchases all personal health services, and contracts with public and private providers on equal terms. The 60 municipalities of Lithuania own a large share of the primary care centres, particularly the polyclinics, and small-to-medium sized hospitals. They are also responsible delivering public health activities.

Service delivery continues to be dominated by a large and mostly public hospitals sector but outpatient service delivery is increasingly mixed. Inpatient services remain mostly publicly provided and the total number of beds, 7 per 1000 population, is well above the OECD average of 4.7. Specialist outpatient care is delivered through the outpatient departments of hospitals or polyclinics, as well as by private providers. Private providers play an increasing role in the rapidly-developing day care and day surgery segment as well as in diagnostic and interventional imaging services. Primary care is provided in either municipality-owned facilities or typically smaller private practices.

Lithuania has more physicians and fewer nurses per capita than the OECD average and their geographic distribution is a concern. Despite emigration of health staff, Lithuania has retained a relatively high number of physicians: 4.3 per 1000 population versus 3.4 in the OECD. The ratio of nurses to population on the other hand is below the OECD average. Specialists, in particular, are unequally distributed across the country. In order to attract staff in peripheral areas, GPs receive a higher capitation payment for patients living in rural areas, and hospitals/municipalities offer higher salaries. In conjunction with municipalities, the government has recently put in place grants for medical students willing to work in remote areas. Overall though, no systematic tools are in place to assess future needs and gaps, or to evaluate the impact of current policies.

An appropriate set of policy directions has been consistently pursued over time

Health features as a prominent inter-sectoral priority across Lithuania's main strategic planning documents. For instance, "Health for All" is one of three horizontal priorities of the country's national development strategy, "Lithuania 2030". The implementation of "Health for All" is governed by a specific intersectoral action plan coordinated by the Ministry of Health and involving nine other Ministries. Another set of inter-ministerial strategy and plans specifically focus on drug, alcohol and tobacco control and prevention. Overall, these documents demonstrate a clear recognition that improving health is important to the development of Lithuania and requires efforts beyond the health sector.

Furthermore stakeholders in Lithuania agree on priorities which are aligned with the burden of disease and reforms which are conducive to achieving these objectives. In particular, reforms have consistently sought to reorganise service delivery by developing primary health care, restructuring the hospital system, modernizing payment systems, and strengthening public health.

The current Lithuanian health strategy is articulated around a life-course approach which emphasises the importance of tackling health determinants and reducing inequalities. The strategy specifically targets the excessive burden of cardio-vascular diseases and recognises the need for additional emphasis on mental health. The programme of the government formed in 2016 is also aligned with these long-standing priorities. In other words, many conditions are met for Lithuania's health system to deliver good results.

Spending on health remains low

Lithuania however, continues to spend little on health despite some convergence with OECD countries. In 2015, expenditure per capita stood at USD 1 883 adjusted for purchasing power parity and represented 6.5% of GDP. For both measures, Lithuania stands in the bottom quintile of the OECD distribution even if, over time, its position has improved.

The structure of spending between different categories of care has also converged towards the OECD average. Lithuania continues to spend relatively more on inpatient care and medical goods and less on outpatient care and long-term care than OECD countries, but the difference is less pronounced than a decade ago. Two thirds of spending in Lithuania is public, which is lower than the OECD average of 73%, a level Lithuania had managed to reach ten years ago.

Despite progress, the health status of the population is poor

Life expectancy is lower than anywhere in the OECD

Life expectancy at birth is six years below the OECD average and in 2015, lower than anywhere in the OECD. Over the past 45 years, Lithuania's accumulated gain in average life expectancy at birth has been less than four years. Moreover, Lithuania is marked by a larger gender gap in life expectancy than in any OECD country and women live nearly 11 years longer than men.

Chronic conditions and external causes contribute most to the life expectancy gap between Lithuania and OECD countries

Chronic conditions account for majority of deaths in Lithuania, followed by external causes (accidents and intentional self-harm). Cardiovascular diseases (CVDs - including ischemic heart disease, stroke and other diseases of circulatory system) are the leading cause of death in Lithuania, accounting for 56% of deaths. Lithuanians die three times more frequently of heart attacks than citizens of the OECD on average. Progress in reducing mortality from CVDs has been slower than in other parts of Eastern Europe: Lithuania, Hungary and Estonia had a comparable mortality in 2003 and while it has decreased by 22% in Lithuania, in Hungary it has declined by 33% and Estonia 56%.

The second leading cause of mortality is cancer – 20% of deaths. While mortality is higher than the OECD average, this rate is closer to the average than in a number of eastern European countries. Accidents and intentional self-harm (suicides) – external causes of mortality – account for 8% of deaths and death rates from external causes, which are much higher among men than women, explain a large part of the gender gap in mortality. Lithuania records in particular the highest rate of mortality from suicide in the OECD. It has decreased by 42% between 1995 and 2015, but is still more than double the OECD average for the general population and nearly three-times the OECD average for men.

Fewer adults in Lithuania report being in good or excellent health than in the OECD on average. Only 43% of the population aged 15 years and above reports good or very good health while the OECD average is 68%. Furthermore, inequalities are high: in 2015, only 32% of Lithuanians in the lowest income quantile reported to be in good or very good health against 63% of the population in the highest income quintile. Elderly people in Lithuania report particularly poor health. Only 6% of the population aged 65 and over reports to be in good or very good health, markedly below the OECD average of 44%. Moreover, the average number of healthy life years at age 65 – an indicator of disability-free life expectancy - is among the lowest in the OECD for both women and men – 5.5 and 5 years, respectively.

Harmful alcohol consumption is the leading risk factor and continues to increase

Harmful alcohol consumption is a major risk factor behind the leading causes of death in Lithuania. Among Lithuanians aged 15 years and above, the consumption of alcohol per capita is significantly higher than in any OECD country and as much as 69% above the OECD average. Alcohol consumption has been on the rise in Lithuania – an opposite trend to that seen in the majority of OECD countries. Youth are particularly vulnerable: among 15-years-olds as many as 41% of boys and 33% of girls in Lithuania reported having been drunk at least twice in their life, which is the highest for boys and the third highest for girls as compared with the European member countries of the OECD in 2013-2014.

Other risk factors, such as tobacco smoking and obesity, are less widespread than alcohol consumption. In 2015, around 20% of Lithuanians aged 15 and over reported to be daily smokers, which is slightly above average of 18% in the OECD, but men in Lithuania are among the top three heaviest smokers in the OECD. Nevertheless, unlike alcohol consumption, regular smoking has been decreasing over the recent decade. Obesity in Lithuania, on the other hand is below the OECD average. Overall, the gender gap in life expectancy can be attributed at least partly to the differences in risky health behaviours.

All in all, a large number of premature deaths could be avoided

Lithuania has among the high rates of avoidable mortality in the EU. Data from Eurostat show that amenable mortality in Lithuania, which captures the number of deaths which could be avoided through better quality care, is 2.5 higher than the EU average. Preventable mortality, which could be avoided through better control of the wider determinants of health, is twice the EU average. In other words, if more effective public health and medical interventions were in place, fewer people would die prematurely in Lithuania.

The production and use of data is increasing but more attention to policy impact is required

Lithuania's already rich data infrastructure continues to expand. Health services providers report on numerous performance indicators to the NHIF, the Ministry of Health and related institutions (although private providers tend to under-report). In many cases, this information is made public and availed to patients in a way which allows them to access it on a facility-by-facility basis. For the first time in 2017, Lithuania reported to the OECD standard health care quality indicators. E-health is being developed and a number of key records, including for instance prescriptions and discharge summaries can be electronically stored and exchanged. In sum, the use e-health is growing and the availability of data is improving.

At the same time, the use of data for performance assessment and decision making remains insufficient. Performance data are not always statistically analysed, rarely presented in dashboards or used for benchmarking progress of entities responsible for delivering results like individual facilities and municipalities. Such tools would support more effective accountability for results. Similarly, progress on reform implementation is systematically monitored but more attention is paid to determining whether activities have been completed compared to their impact. Stakeholders recognise that the resources to analyse results and policy impact are limited. Developing in-house capacity or partnering with outside (academic) institutions, including those who collect data, are options which should be explored.

Sustainability and access

Lithuania's public investment in health is carefully managed and the system so far is on a financially sustainable path

Public spending is comparatively low but was, by and large, protected during the crisis and institutions at all levels are held accountable for budget management

Countries with higher income tend to spend more on health, but even accounting for the fact that Lithuania's income is lower than the OECD average, it spends relatively little on health. The low level of public spending is the result of Lithuania's overall relatively small size of government (public spending represents 35% of GDP compared to an OECD average of 44% in 2015), and the low priority given to health within the public budget: 10% of it is allocated to health when the OECD average is 15%.

Yet, the public health financing architecture in place proved to be remarkably resilient in the face of the major financial crisis of 2009 and in this respect, Lithuania is widely recognised as a good practice example. The NHIF is predominantly funded through contributions from the employed, which in 2016 represented 73% of its revenues. In addition, the NHIF receives a transfer from the general budget which corresponds to a fixed amount per inactive person statutorily covered. During the crisis, this mechanism was instrumental in protecting health spending: as revenues collected from the active population dropped sharply, transfers from the state increased with the increased number of unemployed. The share of general budget funding in NHIF revenue rose from less than 20% before the crisis to around 35% between 2010 and 2013 before returning to its current level of 27%.

Budget management procedures are effective at keeping public spending in check. By law, the NHIF must balance revenues and expenditure each year. In each budget cycle, it sets aside provisions to adjust payments to service providers based on the services actually delivered at the end of the year. The NHIF also builds up reserves which can be used in case of revenue shortages or unexpected expenditure increases. They served as a buffer during the financial crisis and have also been used to increase tariffs and compensate facilities for increases in the base salary of health workers decided by the Ministry. In contrast to a number of countries in the region where public facilities are often in deficit and accumulate debts, the finances of public institutions delivering health services are generally financially sound.

The system so far is on a financial sustainable path but additional investment must be strategically managed

So far, Lithuania's health system is on a financially sustainable path. As seen above, Lithuania's spending is on the low side and from a public finance perspective, kept in check. Additionally, Lithuania's health expenditure is not projected to grow as quickly as that of other EU members. Under the reference scenario of the 2013-2060 European Commission projections, Lithuania, along with Belgium, is one of the two countries with the lowest anticipated growth in public health expenditure among EU countries (0.1 p.p. over the period). The overall picture is thus one of financial sustainability.

Recent decisions though envisage significant increases in salaries for health workers. In 2016, the salaries of all staff working in health institutions increased by 8% and in 2017, a further 8% increase was granted to nurses and physicians. An agreement was reached in 2017 between Trade Unions and the Ministry of Health to implement a further 20% rise in 2018 for all staff working in health institutions. Finally, fairly ambitious targets were set for health workers salaries in relation to the average wage in the economy to be reached by 2020. Blanket salary increases need to be sustainably funded and attention must be paid to ensuring they do not undermine the resources available for the other inputs or investments the system requires to provide quality services.

So, while consideration should be given to increasing public funding for health in Lithuania, additional investments should also be leveraged to improve the performance of the health system as whole. There is no doubt that some pressure exists to increase salaries in the hope to retain staff to work in the health sector in Lithuania. Relative levels of remuneration across countries can play a role in staff retention, but are not the only element. Overall, a more in depth analysis of the labour market dynamics for health workers in Lithuania should be undertaken and a comprehensive strategy devised to address current and future human resources imbalances more systematically. More broadly, blanket salary increases should not be the only driver of public health spending. Additional public funding is necessary to improve the population's health outcomes and financial protection, but investments should be targeted to the amenable burden of diseases and based on evidence of effectiveness.

Despite significant out-of-pocket payments, access to services is broadly adequate

Coverage is broad but household still face high out-of-pocket payments

The population is adequately covered by the public health insurance scheme managed by the NHIF. All citizens and legal residents are required to seek coverage from the NHIF and the vast majority comply. The state guarantees coverage for the economically inactive and the estimated 2% to 4% of the population which is uninsured is entitled to free emergency care. Coverage is quite broad but patient co-payments apply on most outpatient medicines. In fact, the co-payment rules for medicine are complex and result from co-insurance but also the fact that patients who do not choose the cheapest medicine in a group of presumed comparable ones (for instance, a generic), pay the difference out-of-pocket.

In 2015, out of pocket payments represented around 32% of health spending in Lithuania, among the highest levels in the OECD where the average is 20%. Private health insurance is not developed in Lithuania, thus the bulk of private spending is out of pocket (OOP). The proportion of health expenditure paid OOP was around 33% in the mid-2000s, decreasing somewhat during the financial crisis due to a sharp reduction in private relative to public spending growth rates, and has risen again after 2012. Out-of-pocket payments represent 40% of spending on ambulatory services and 68% of the cost of medicines and medical goods, on par with Latvia which is the highest of the OECD (where the average is 42%).

Out-of-pocket spending has an impoverishing effect on part of the population. WHO suggests that the risk of impoverishment from OOP costs becomes significant in countries where these represent more than 20% of total spending. A forthcoming WHO report on Lithuania showed that in 2012 (most recent year for which data is available) 9.4% of the population experienced financial hardship due to health spending, a reduction from the 2008 level of 11.5% but higher than in 2005 (7%). The incidence of catastrophic spending is heavily concentrated among older people (those aged 60 and over) and couples without children. Eighty percent of catastrophic spending is due to medicines, and this proportion is even higher among households belonging to the lowest income quintile.

A number of steps have been taken in 2017 to try to curb out-of-pocket payments on medicines and increase the transparency of pharmaceutical policy. These include a reduction in the VAT on expensive medicines and caps put on the difference between the prices at which medicines are offered in pharmacies and their reference prices (to which the reimbursement rates by the NHIF apply). Consideration is also being given to developing a separate model for the reimbursement of medicines for low-income patients. Additional measures aim to promote the use of generics and the rational use of medicines. Many of these measures were outlined in Lithuania's first medicines policy guidelines, adopted by the government in 2017. The guidelines also included other intentions, in particular, the strengthening of Health Technology Assessment in collaboration with other countries. This represents are a promising step in the direction of more effective policies whose progress and impact should be monitored.

Informal payments were widespread in Lithuania but recent data suggest they might be declining. Informal payments seem to have been more widespread in Lithuania than in comparable countries. A 2013 Transparency International report, based on a survey implemented in a range of countries, inquired whether people had paid a bribe when accessing services. In Lithuania, 35% declared having done so, by far the highest proportion in the OECD where the average was 7%. In 2015, the Ministry of Health put a strategy in place to tackle informal payments, which is currently under implementation. The most recent data suggest that informal payments may be decreasing. In the 2017 Eurobarometer on corruption, only 12% of people who had been in contact with the system in the previous year declared having made a non-official fee or gift to the doctor, nurse or hospital, when in 2013 the proportion in the same survey was 21%.

Key metrics nevertheless suggest access to care is adequate in Lithuania

Compared with OECD averages, people in Lithuania access health services frequently. In 2016, individuals consulted physicians on average 8.8 times a year, nearly 20% above the OECD average. Around two thirds of these visits were to primary care physicians (NHIF data). In 2015 there was an average of 24 hospital discharges per 1000 population. This is the third highest discharge rate among OECD countries and 50% above the average. This suggests that access to services is not constrained.

Unmet needs are comparatively lower than in other similar countries. In the 25 EU countries of the OECD, on average, 3.2% of the population declared not having sought care for financial, geographic or waiting time reasons in 2015, compared with 2.9% in Lithuania. In addition, in most countries where the proportion of the population foregoing care exceeds 2%, individuals in low income households are much more likely than those in high income households to do so. In Lithuania, this difference is relatively small.

Few Lithuanians perceive financial barriers to access. In Lithuania, only 2% of the population declared having foregone medical care for financial reasons in the 2014 European Health Interview Survey. The proportion foregoing dental care was 5%, but only 2% for prescribed pharmaceuticals, which is surprising given the extensive out-of-pocket payments on medicines. Relatively speaking, waiting times are much more of a constraint to access. Three-quarters of the people declaring having foregone medical care do so because of waiting times (SILC 2015). This represents 2% of the population, significantly above the 1% EU28 average but nevertheless below the United Kingdom (2.5%), Finland (4.2%) and Estonia (above 11%).

Increasing attention will need to be paid to measuring and, as needed, addressing possible barriers in access to care. While high-level analyses suggest access to care in Lithuania is reasonable, a more nuanced understanding of the situation is required. Indeed, available data are not sufficiently detailed to assess the nature and the distribution of the financial burden people face in accessing care and particularly in obtaining medicines. Little is known about the constraints faced by those living in rural areas. While summary data on waiting times are not readily available it is likely that access to care is problematic for some groups of the population and may contribute to inequalities in outcomes. Monitoring systems need to be strengthened and measures designed to address identified issues.

On balance, the overall assessment of the performance of Lithuania's health system on the key dimensions of sustainability and access is rather positive. Lithuania's spending on health is low and efforts to keep public spending in check are effective. At the same time, the sustainability of the system is not only a matter of public finance. Improving health outcomes and the financial protection of the population is likely to require additional investments. Nevertheless, people have reasonable access to the system and unmet needs are lower than in countries with comparable income and spending. This balance – as everywhere – is a difficult one to maintain. In particular, more needs to be done to protect people from high out-of-pocket spending on pharmaceuticals and to ensure that additional funds invested in the system are geared towards improving the health of the population. As the next section will show, efforts in particular will need to be stepped up to increase the efficiency and quality of services delivered.

Efficiency and quality

Comparative studies have shown that several European countries and OECD economies with a level of income and health spending comparable to those of Lithuania achieve considerably higher life expectancy. Put differently, these high-level analyses suggest significant scope for improving the efficiency and quality, in particular the effectiveness, of service delivery in Lithuania and resonate with the fact that both preventable and amenable mortality are high compared to other European countries.

Efforts in rebalancing service delivery must be pursued and deepened to increase efficiency

Prior to 1990, the role of primary health care and health promotion was limited and services were predominantly delivered in a range of hospitals, which were numerous and frequently narrowly specialized by disease or population segment. Reorganising the hospital sector and reducing its size, rebalancing service delivery in favour of a modernised and considerably strengthened primary care and developing better strategies to tackle risk factors have been the main drivers behind service delivery reforms in Eastern and central Europe since transition. Lithuania is no exception and all stakeholders have been consistently aligned behind these priorities.

Lithuania's steady efforts to overhaul the hospital sector need to be pursued

The current configuration of the hospital system represents significant progress in shaping the hospital sector. In 2015, there were 119 public hospitals, significantly less than the 202 in 1991. The number of monoprofile hospitals has substantially decreased. The MoH manages 10 "republican level" facilities and there are 49 smaller municipal hospitals. Since 1992, more than half of the beds have been closed through administratively planned downsizing and application of incentives such as shifting the funding to an output based reimbursement.

Still, many countries have been more effective in consolidating hospital infrastructure. Today Lithuania remains with Germany, Austria and Hungary among the European countries with the most hospital beds. Compared to neighbouring Baltic countries, the pace of change in reducing hospital capacity has been relatively slow: between 2000 and 2015, the number of beds in Latvia dropped by 54%, in Estonia by 42% and in Lithuania by 27%.

Average lengths of stay are relatively short but the low and very variable bed occupancy rate indicates the hospital sector remains in overcapacity. In 2015, among the 65 public general hospitals, the average bed occupancy rate was 73.5%, which is below the OECD average of 77%. There are however large variations among general hospitals with predominantly small hospitals reporting very low rates. The current health system development plan aims to increased bed occupancy levels and sets a target of 300 days per year (above 82%). In 2015, only 4 of the 65 public general hospitals in Lithuania met this target. In fact, the bed occupancy rate was lower than 60% in 13 public hospitals.

Payment systems and contracting methods have been increasingly leveraged to encourage more efficient modes of delivery

Diagnosis-related group-based payments (DRG) combined with volume caps seek to encourage efficient use of resources and lower volumes of inpatient hospitalisations. In 2012, a DRG system based on the Australian coding and diagnosis grouping was introduced and continues to be fine-tuned. To account for the fact that DRG systems can encourage increases in the number of hospitalisations, contracts between the NHIF with individual facilities include volume ceilings for in-patient services which are decreased year-on-year.

Contracting and payments have also effectively encouraged the development of day-cases and outpatient surgery. Day-cases are paid at the full DRG price. In addition, for individual hospitals, day-cases volumes are not capped. Among the 71 main procedures eligible to be performed as day-cases, the proportion actually performed as day-cases was 58% in 2016, an increase of 20 percentage points compared with 2012. In 2016, tonsillectomies were included in the day-case list and around 45% were performed as day cases that same year. In other words, hospitals are actively developing the day-case activity.

Further consolidation of service delivery is warranted on efficacy and safety grounds and steps have been taken in that direction

Surgeries are undertaken in the vast majority of hospitals in Lithuania, which is inefficient and also carries a risk for patients. Of the 65 hospitals with a general profile contracted by the NHIF, 52 provided at least one surgical procedure in a 12 month period (2015 data). Among them, 22 carried out less than 250 procedures, which is roughly one per (business) day. Moreover, the number and complexity of these procedures varies considerably across hospitals, and many carry out major surgeries which could be programmed at very low frequency. Concentrating their delivery in a few places could allow a more efficient use of staff and equipment. More importantly, the fact that so many facilities carry out few surgeries raises serious concerns about their capacity to deliver good outcomes.

A recent decision to use minimum volume thresholds for contracting is a bold step in the right direction. Lithuania intends on concentrating services in fewer places and is using volume targets for obstetrics and common surgeries in contracting to that effect. Since 2016, the plan is that unless a hospital is more than 50km away from the nearest one, or it has recently received specific investments, it will no longer be contracted by the NHIF when if carries out fewer than 300 births per year or less than 400 major surgeries. In 2015, half of the public general hospitals in Lithuania (31 of 65) had an obstetric department. In 14 of these, less than 300 deliveries were conducted.

Further restructuring may also require planning and organising service delivery at a higher level of government. The reconfiguration of hospital service delivery is difficult in all countries. Progress in Lithuania has been hampered by the fact that municipalities, which own and manage hospitals, have a natural tendency to protect local interests, in terms of perceived access to services or simply employment. Many countries in the wider Europe region have realised that the distribution of hospitals services needs to be decided at a higher level than the municipality and reverted to more central planning including Finland, Austria, Denmark and Croatia.

Primary care is modern and well organised

Lithuania clearly recognises that a strong primary health care is the foundation of a health system that is effective, efficient and responsive to patients' needs and has developed the system accordingly.

The introduction and development of family medicine were encouraged early on and today, the number of GPs per population is higher in Lithuania than in most OECD countries. Primary care is delivered by teams which must include a nurse, who is being given increasing autonomy and responsibilities in the management of chronic patients with non-communicable diseases. The number of PHC visits per person per year has increased from 4.8 in 2007 to 5.7 in 2014.

Primary care services are delivered in a variety of public and private settings remunerated through a mixed but predominantly capitation-based system. Most PHC facilities are owned by the municipalities but private clinics can open and work on the same terms as public ones. In cities, polyclinics also include outpatient specialists. In remote areas public facilities can also run community medical dispensaries to bring services closer to the population. Public facilities are typically larger entities: they represent 39% of PHC providers but cover around 70% of the population. Public and private providers are all contracted and monitored the same way. A little less than three quarters of their remuneration comes from a capitation adjusted for age and they receive additional payments to incentivise quality.

Primary care providers have been given a key role in managing patients' health. Virtually the entire population is registered with a GP or a primary care team. Patients cannot obtain free PHC services unless they are registered with a GP and referrals are required for specialised care in most cases. PHC providers are financially incentivised to deliver specific services and expected to coordinate patient care. They must also be informed about care provided by others (specialists, hospitals). PHC providers are required to ensure access to care 24/7. Compared to other EU countries, a smaller share of emergency department visitors report they did so due to unavailability of primary care.

GPs' role could be further strengthened in some areas, on efficiency but also quality grounds. The delineation of responsibilities between GPs and specialist needs to further evolve and GPs believe that some guidelines continue to unnecessarily limit their responsibilities. Primary care teams also need to play an increasing role in the coordination of their patients' care as well as in mental health.

Renewed efforts to strengthen public health policies must be sustained

The main challenges with regard to the state of public health are well recognised. The populations' health status and behaviours indicate sizeable room for improvement. The 2014-2025 Lithuanian Health Strategy specifies concrete goals with regard to reducing harmful alcohol consumption, tobacco, drugs and psychoactive substances, as well as encouraging healthy nutrition and physical activity. The Strategy has an impressive cross-sectorial framework (involving nearly all Ministries), and the MoH is responsible for monitoring of the implementation. Intermediate evaluation of the progress is due in 2020.

In recent years, Lithuania has introduced additional measures to tackle the exceptionally high alcohol consumption. The Parliament has adopted a number of evidence-based alcohol control measures, such as restrictions on alcohol advertising and on alcohol selling hours, as we as a prohibition to sell alcohol in the gas stations. Lithuania also raised most alcohol excise rates in March 2017 substantially, e.g. from 336 to 711 Euros per hectolitre pure alcohol on beer (MoH). In June 2017, additional alcohol restrictions were approved, which came into effect 1st of January 2018. From this date, Lithuania has a full ban on alcohol advertisement on TV, radio and internet. Alcohol sales hours were shortened, and the minimum legal age for buying and consuming alcoholic beverages was raised to 20 years.

These steps are all welcome and Lithuania should carefully monitor and evaluate the enforcement level of these policies. Additional gains in health and life expectancy can be obtained through interventions targeting heavy drinkers as well as drug and psychosocial therapy of alcohol dependence, which, along with worksite-based interventions, are effective and have favourable cost-effectiveness profiles in the long run.

In general, evidence that highly effective public health interventions are actively pursued is limited at all levels. There have been few concrete initiatives. At the local level, the responsibility for public health mainly lies with municipalities, who are encouraged to set up and run (or contract if they do not have one) Public Health Bureaus (currently 47 across 60 municipalities). However, municipalities are for the most part free to choose the activities they implement and decide on their level of effort. No framework is in place to help ensure that local-level stakeholders implement evidence-based interventions or are accountable for progress on results (as opposed to simply implementation).

Overall, many public health efforts are geared towards small initiatives which are insufficiently evaluated. Most interventions, such as information sessions on harmful alcohol use or benefits of healthy diet at the Public Health Bureaus, are assessed in terms of process indicators, such as a number of participants, and not focused on outcomes. Project design, including monitoring and evaluation, must focus also on the effectiveness of these actions. This could improve results, which have been below expectation in many programs, notably those targeting harmful alcohol consumption.

Further priority can be given to increased and stable funding for public health services. Lithuania allocates 1.9% (2016) of health spending to preventive services, noticeably below the OECD average. Many initiatives and research projects are conducted within time-limited EU funded projects. While project-based testing and piloting is good to find effective approaches, there is a risk that many good projects will not be sustained without a more robust financing framework for these functions.

More attention must be paid to improving the quality of care

Lithuania has put in place a number of initiatives to support improvements in quality of care

Key policies and institutions to improve quality of care are in place. The State Health Care Accreditation Agency has long been responsible for licensing of health care organisations and most professionals and has launched an accreditation program in 2016. However, by the end of 2016, only five PHC organisations had applied for accreditation and ten more were in the preparation stage. In January 2017 a financial incentive in the form of a marginally higher capitation for accredited clinics was introduced, although it seems to be inadequate to substantially raise interest. By the end of 2017 only 16 institutions were accredited.

Some clinical guidelines exist but information about their effective use lacking. The Ministry of Health has issued 123 diagnostic and treatment protocols (in cardiology, oncology, neurology, traumatology and paediatrics). Providers are encouraged and supposed to follow them, regardless of the ownership or level and volume of the services provided but no mechanisms are in place to monitor compliance or support providers in implementation. To date, patient safety has received very little attention. Overall, Lithuania lacks a system-wide support for continuous health care quality improvement at the clinical level.

A number of recent initiatives put greater emphasis on measuring and – at least for primary care – rewarding quality.

Quality is increasingly monitored and Lithuania in 2017 reported data on a range of OECD-HCQI indicators. In 2012, a set of 15 quality indicators for hospitals was adopted, in line with the PATH (Performance Assessment Tool for Quality Improvement in Europe) recommendations. However, the procedure for engaging hospitals in a quality discussion, limited to a yearly discussion of the results between the managers of the facilities and the NHIF, is weak. For primary care, a set of indicators is used to calculate a performance-based add-on to the capitation.

Information on quality is shared transparently in an effort to support informed choices by patients. Quality indicators for hospitals are published annually. For primary care, many quality indicators are calculated to facilitate bench marking by clinics and municipalities. For patients, data on individual facilities' performance is readily available on-line, published by the five territorial insurance funds. While this is a very welcome step towards improving transparency, further steps could be taken to contextualise and make this information user-friendly.

PHC remuneration is organised to reward performance, through fees for services and a pay-for-performance component. Facilities receive an age and sex-adjusted capitation rate (72.9% of total PHC facilities' revenue in 2016) with an additional per capita amount for rural facilities (7.1% of revenue). PHC providers also receive activity- or output-based payments for a list of specific services (10.7% of revenue). The final element of remuneration is a result-based payment based on a list of performance indicators (9.3% of revenue).

The performance based payment for PHC is well intended and monitored, and some indicators show improvements although from low levels. Twelve indicators are taken into account to determine the payment. They include to the proportion of registered adults and children who visits the clinic at least once per year, rates of cancer screening and rates of hospitalisations of patients with chronic diseases. Results are monitored by the NHIF, which for instance show that the cervical cancer screening rate for registered patients rose from 23% in 2008 to 35% in 2015.

While the focus of the pay-for-performance scheme on non-communicable diseases is welcome, a review and revision would be warranted to better encourage the delivery of appropriate services. For example, a high share of listed adults who visit PHC over one year, which generates a bonus payment, does not necessarily mean the clinic meets those in most need of a consultation. Furthermore, general check-ups for healthy adults are not shown to improve morbidity or mortality. Finally, access in Lithuania is well developed and in 2016, 92% of PHC clinics reached the highest level of performance on this indicator. Therefore, the usefulness of this indicator in the performance scheme could – at this point – be debated. As another example, the indicators on avoidable hospitalisations which are certainly relevant to monitor the performance of PHC at a high level, may not be so appropriate at the level of a single (especially small) facility as they are not only impacted by primary care. For chronic diseases, performance schemes more typically use processes indicators to reward clinical excellence (for example, blood pressure checks for patients with hypertension, tests for HgbA1c for diabetic patient) or better intermediate outcomes (for example, cholesterol control in people with diabetes or controlled blood pressure). So, while monitoring and rewarding performance may be appropriate, the current system could be better calibrated.

Two interesting initiatives to strengthen specific services which have a strong potential to increase the effectiveness of service delivery and thus quality have recently been introduced.

First, an EU-funded programme supporting the integration of health and social services encourages care co-ordination. In 2013, the Ministry of Social Security and Labour launched the Integrated Assistance Programme to offer integrated health and social care to the disabled and elderly. In 21 municipalities, 70 mobile teams provide integrated services (nursing and social care) at home, including support to their informal care givers. Funding from the EU will support the expansion to all municipalities but funding is only secured until 2020. The project-based approach can help devise effective solutions to integrate services, but carry a risk that they may not be sustained. Given the increasing population need for such services, the program should be carefully evaluated and – if cost-effective – sustainably funded.

Second, the recently introduced functional clustering can strengthen the quality of specific hospital services for which rapid access is needed. In 2013, standardised pathways were introduced for stroke and myocardial infarction with elevated ST, conditions for which a fast response is required. Depending on severity, patients are directed by emergency services either to the regional hospital or one of the six regional stroke treatment centres or five cardiology centres established by the program. For strokes, the program has allowed the development of intravenous (IV) thrombolysis or thrombectomy in the country, two types of procedures used to treat and remove blood clots from the body. The rates of IV thrombolysis, a quality indicator monitored in stroke care which remains disappointingly low in many high income countries has increased dramatically in Lithuania. In 2012, 160 intravenous thrombolyses were performed while in 2016, 808 were performed. For thrombectomies the number rose from 4 to 276 in that same period. These measures, as well as selective contracting based on minimum volume, hold great potential for increasing the quality of inpatient services in Lithuania but it will be critical to demonstrate more rigorously that they lead to improvements in clinical outcomes.

Despite progress, quality of care indicators still place Lithuania among OECD's poor performers

Survey data consistently shows that patients in Lithuania are more satisfied with services than a few years ago. For instance, according to Eurobarometer, the population's view on the quality of health care improved dramatically between 2009 and 2013. Between these 4 years, the share of Lithuanians rating the overall quality of health care in the country as good increased from 40 to 65%, the largest increase among European Union countries, although this share is still below the EU average (71%). However, measures of clinical outcomes show that progress is required at all levels.

Prevention and treatment at the primary care level can still improve. For instance, immunisation rates could be higher. High rates of children immunisation were one of the hallmarks of soviet systems, which many countries have retained. Results in this regard in Lithuania are a bit disappointing being around or slightly below OECD averages. Although Influenza vaccination coverage for people above 65 is much higher than in Latvia and Estonia, at 19.5% it also remains well below the OECD average of 43% in 2015.

PHC in Lithuania is increasingly effective in managing chronic diseases and keeping people out of the hospital. Hospitalisations for ambulatory care sensitive conditions are among the key quality indicators for primary care. Hospitalisations for these conditions have been declining in Lithuania since 2005, although from very high starting levels. In fact, for Asthma and COPD, the rates are converging with OECD averages. However, this progress is only relative as many countries manage to achieve substantially lower rates of hospitalisations. On the other hand, despite progress, for congestive heart failure, the proportion of patients hospitalised still remains the highest among 32 countries reporting this indicator to the OECD, more than twice the average rate. Hospitalisation rates for diabetes are a third higher than the OECD average and do not seem to decline.

Hospital mortality for acute conditions is also stubbornly high. Mortality after hospitalisation for acute conditions is the most common indicator for measuring hospital care quality and is collected by the OECD for international comparison purposes. For the first time, Lithuania provided 30 day mortality data for acute myocardial infarction, haemorrhagic stroke and ischemic stroke in 2017. In all cases, Lithuania's figures considerably exceed OECD averages. For instance, Lithuania has the second highest mortality rates compared to OECD countries that are able to link mortality data across health providers for AMI and ischaemic stroke. Although Lithuanian data is only available for four years (2012–2015), results have not improved over this period. This reinforces the recommendation to monitor the impact of on-going clustering of stroke and cardiac services. In addition, Lithuania should expand the number of quality indicators reported to the OECD, particularly on patient safety to better benchmark its performance.

Cancer offers a disease-oriented and systemic perspective on quality as results depend on both effective PHC and hospital services. Despite progress, PHC providers struggle to ensure better coverage of cancer screening. Lithuania has set up publicly funded population-based screening programs for common cancers: breast, prostate, colorectal and cervical cancer and coverage of the target population has increased over the last 10 years. For instance, in 2015, 45% of targeted women had been screened for breast cancer compared to only 12% in 2006, a significant improvement from very low levels but still below the OECD average of 61%.

Overall, the effectiveness of cancer care quality has improved considerably but still lags behind most OECD countries. Five-year survival rates after cancer diagnosis for most forms of cancer have increased substantially over the past decade and faster than in many other countries, but remain among the lowest in the OECD. Breast cancer survival has increased from 65% to 74% between 2000–04 to 2010–14, but it remains behind those of neighbouring Baltic countries Latvia and Estonia. Similarly colorectal cancer treatment is increasingly successful and at par with neighbouring countries. Colon cancer survival has increased from 45% to 57% in the same time period (CONCORD programme, LSHTM, 2018). For prostate cancer, survival has doubled between the late 1990s and the late 2000s. However, much of the increase in cancer survival is driven by earlier detection, which increases survival also without decreasing mortality (Krilaviciute et al., 2014). All in all thus, from diagnostic to treatment, progress is still needed.

To summarise, there remains room to improve the efficiency and quality in the Lithuanian health system. Progress in restructuring the hospital sector has been slower than in other countries and many facilities still perform very few surgeries and deliveries, which is inefficient but also detrimental to quality and carries a risk for patients. The ongoing initiatives to cluster services in fewer hospitals, and develop a small number of specialised hospitals for some conditions, are promising but need to be extended, sustained over a long time frame and their impact evaluated.

PHC is well organised and reflects best OECD practices and several indicators suggest that PHC has a positive impact on wider system efficiency, as shown by the decreasing hospitalisations for ambulatory care sensitive conditions. However, the coverage of preventive services, in particular cancer screening, is still disappointing. Coordination with public health and mental health services has been on the agenda for some time but results are still modest. Curbing unhealthy behaviours, such as harmful drinking and smoking, particularly among men, is essential to closing the gap with high performing OECD countries.

Overall, the focus on quality needs to be strengthened in Lithuania. The quality assurance culture remains underdeveloped and the policies to change this have not yet been effective. Measuring results and holding stakeholders more explicitly accountable for results can contribute to strengthening clinical outcomes.

Key recommendations

This chapter concludes with key recommendations which could help improve Lithuania's health system performance.

Key Policy Recommendations

Lithuania's health system has many elements in place to ensure comprehensive and equitable access to good quality care. More decisive action is however needed on a number of fronts.

Sustainability and access

- Strengthen efforts to measure and understand limitations to access, in particular due to out-of-pocket payments on pharmaceuticals, informal payments and for populations living in remote areas, and develop appropriate policies.
- Monitor and address current and future human resources imbalances more systematically.
- Consider increasing public funding for health but ensure investments are targeted to the amenable burden of diseases and intervention based on evidence of effectiveness.
- Ensure that Health Technology Assessment becomes an integrated part of decision making within the health system and continue exploring opportunities for international collaboration in this domain and for procurement.
- Put in place measures promoting the rational use of medicines and encouraging all stakeholders to use generics more systematically.
- Further debate, elaborate and operationalise the principles laid out in the 2017 medicines policy guidelines to address individual and collective affordability, technical and allocative efficiency, and long-term sustainability.

Efficiency and quality

- Continue to strengthen primary care service by developing PHC teams' competencies to deliver effective services including primary and secondary prevention interventions and monitor compliance with clinical guidelines.
- Increase the capacity of the primary care system to recognise, treat and manage common mental disorders and increase access to psychological treatments.
- Develop linkages between PHC and other parts of the system, including hospital and social care, especially for chronic and high-need patients.
- Develop, fund, and implement a comprehensive evidence-based public health and prevention strategy, targeting determinants of health as well as high risk individuals. In particular, develop the evaluation of interventions and projects, and create funding mechanisms which can support sustainable implementation of those successful. Increase the accountability of all stakeholders for delivering results.
- Monitor the effectiveness of implementation of newly introduced policies aimed at reducing harmful alcohol consumption as well as their impact.

- Continue implementing contracting for hospital services based on minimum volumes and ensure the development of a graded and safe hospital-based service delivery.
- Further rationalise hospital delivery and downsize the network. This will require (i) a more formal national service plan to be formulated and (ii) adapting the governance and ownership framework to enable and incentivise reorganisation of service delivery across municipal and possibly regional boundaries. Monitor and evaluate impact as efforts are continued to ensure progress and demonstrate the legitimacy of the change.
- Continue efforts to measure quality objectively, in line with the 2017 effort to report data on OECD's Health Care Quality Indicators, and hold people more accountable for it for instance by developing more systematic benchmarking. Develop formats and channels for disseminating performance data more effectively to both clinicians and patients for primary care providers, and consider expanding it in hospitals.
- Strengthen the quality assurance architecture and develop a continuous quality assurance culture. In particular develop a national adverse event reporting and learning system, and set up a system to encourage and monitor compliance with guidelines.

Governance

- Advance the development of e-health infrastructure, create additional incentives for providers and users to join and use it and pay additional attention to ensuring it is user-friendly.
- Use Lithuania's already rich data more systematically to analyse and hold stakeholders accountable for performance.

Chapter 1. Overview of Lithuania's health care needs and health care system

Following a brief introduction to Lithuania's economic and demographic context, this chapter assesses the health status of the population. The chapter also presents the main features of Lithuania's health system and its governance. The health status of the population in Lithuania remains relatively poor by the OECD standards. The prevalence of unhealthy behaviours, such as alcohol drinking, is particularly high and a considerable share of premature death could be avoided. Spending on health is low, but the health system is overall well poised to tackle these challenges more effectively. The National Health Insurance Fund provides quasi-universal coverage to the population and contracts public and private providers. Most institutional elements of well-performing systems are in place and there is a remarkable consensus of stakeholders behind priorities which are aligned with the burden of disease and reforms which are conducive to tackling them. Strengthening data-driven performance assessment and decision making is key to improving policy impact.

The statistical data for Israel are supplied by and under the responsibility of the relevant Israeli authorities. The use of such data by the OECD is without prejudice to the status of the Golan Heights, East Jerusalem and Israeli settlements in the West Bank under the terms of international law.

Introduction

This chapter presents the socio-economic and demographic context of Lithuania and describes the health status of the population. It presents the main features of the health system and outlines its governance framework.

Lithuania has a dynamic economy and aging population (1.1) in a relatively poor health (1.2). Health spending is low by OECD standards but the overall spending structure has been converging with OECD averages (1.3). The health system has been profoundly transformed since the restoration of independence in 1990 (1.4) and improving health is a consistently stated priority (1.5).

1.1. Lithuania has a dynamic economy and an aging population

Lithuania' economy is currently fast-growing but prone to shocks (1.1.1). Its population is fast aging (1.1.2)

1.1.1. The economy is very dynamic but growth has not been inclusive enough

Lithuania, with 2.9 million inhabitants, is a small but dynamic and open economy, member of the European Union (EU) since 2004 and the Euro Zone since 2015. After the collapse of the central planning system in 1991, Lithuania experienced a difficult but fast transition to market economy. In 1991 and 1992, the country's real annual GDP growth dropped by 6% and 21%, respectively. Yet, Lithuania subsequently became one of the fastest growing economies compared to the OECD (Figure 1.1), and the gap in GDP per capita to the OECD average shrank from 70% in 1993 to around 30% in 2014. Economic growth was accompanied by a rise in living standards reflecting better job opportunities and education, in particular.

Nevertheless, the economy has been vulnerable to external shocks. The Russian financial crisis in 1997-98 was the catalyst for a temporary slowdown and the impact of the global financial crisis of 2008 was severe, with a nearly 15% drop in GDP and unemployment surging up to 18% in 2009. Between 2011 and 2014 economic growth has been again one of the highest among European as well as OECD countries, reflecting a swift recovery from the global financial crisis thanks to the economy's high flexibility (OECD, 2016a). GDP growth slowed in 2015 (to 1.8%) as exports were affected by the recession in Russia and counter-sanctions but it picked up to 2.1% in 2016, and is expected to strengthen in 2017-18 (OECD2016b).

Despite the impressive progress, Lithuania still faces serious challenges such as high income inequality, and a large share of population at risk of poverty. The Gini index – a coefficient that measures income inequality in a society and ranges from 0 (perfect equality) to 100 (maximum inequality) – stood at 37.3 in 2014, well above both the OECD and the EU28 average (OECD Income Distribution and Poverty database, 2016). The share of the population at risk of poverty is the third highest compared to the European member countries of the OECD (Figure 1.2). The poverty is also deep-rooted as the income of the poor is on average 23% below the poverty line.

Figure 1.1. Lithuania has one of the fastest growing economies in the OECD

Average annual real GDP and real GDP per capita growth - Lithuania and OECD countries, 2006 -2015

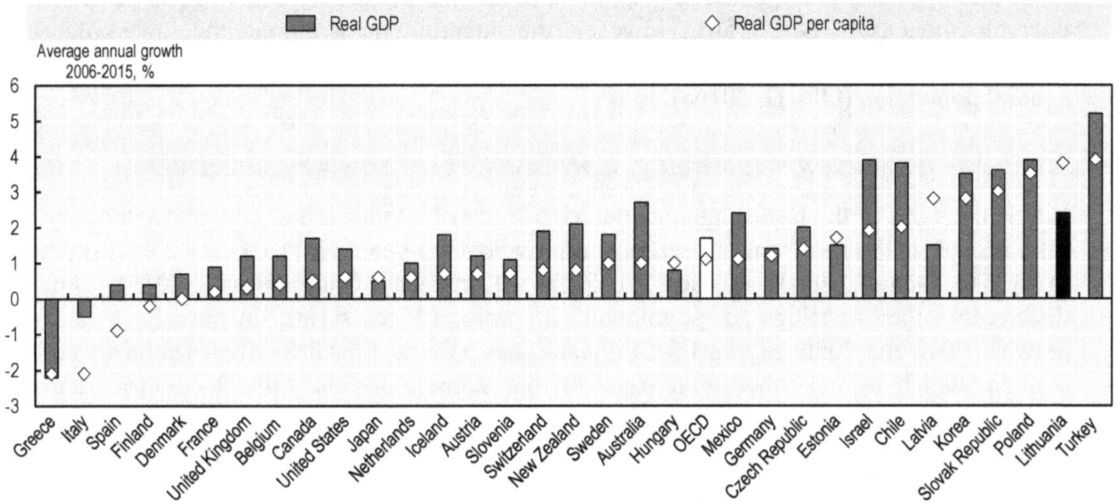

Note: In Lithuania and other Baltic countries GDP per capita grew faster than GDP because of population decline.
Source: OECD (2017a), *OECD Economic Outlook, Volume 2017 Issue 1,* http://dx.doi.org/10.1787/eco_outlook-v2017-1-en.

Figure 1.2. More than 20% of the population is at risk of poverty

Population at risk of poverty, Lithuania and EU28 countries, 2016 (or latest available year).

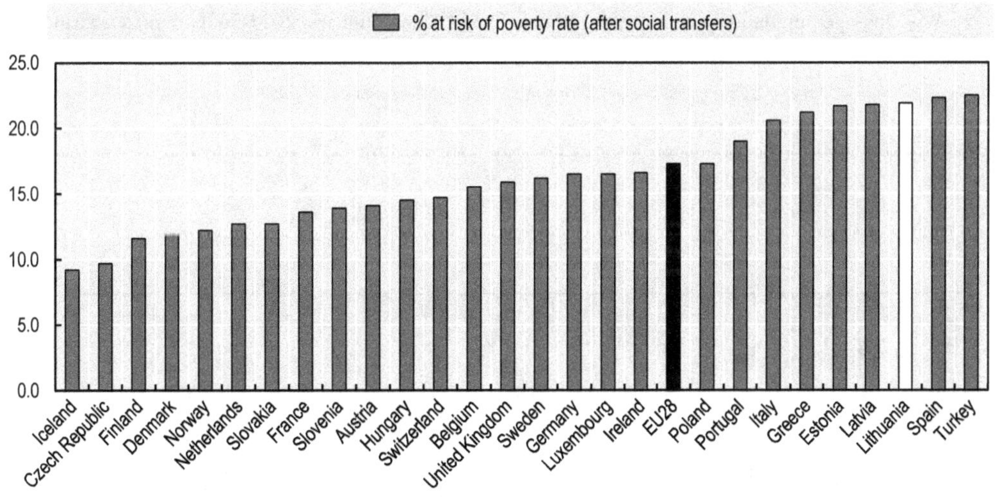

Note: Cut-off point: 60% of median equivalised income after.
Source: Eurostat Population and Social Conditions database, 2017.

Moreover, the unemployment rate of 7.9% (2016) remains above the OECD average of 6.5% (2015), with a nearly 45% share of long-term unemployment. Lithuania's labour market was heavily affected by the global financial crisis, but recovered quickly - the unemployment rate has fallen by two percentage points a year on average since 2010. The unemployment rate for youth, which peaked at 35.7% in 2010, fell to 19.3% in 2014 thanks to specific support measures including training, wage subsidies and a "youth guarantee" which ensures that all youth under 29 get a good-quality offer for a job, training or continued education within four months of leaving education or entering unemployment (OECD, 2015b). However, the unemployment among the low-skilled, which account for majority of the poor, is nearly three times higher than among the general population (OECD, 2016a).

1.1.2. The population is fast aging, a process largely driven by emigration

Lithuania is one of the fastest-ageing countries in the EU. Indeed, the old-age dependency ratio is expected to rise from one senior (person above 65 years old) for every 2.4 workers in 2014 to 1 senior for 1.2 workers in 2050 (European Commission, 2015). Put differently, the working-age population is projected to shrink by nearly a half between 2014 and 2050 (Figure 1.3). Lithuania has a modest fertility rate – 1.6 births per women, which is, nevertheless at par with the average for the OECD countries and slightly higher than in the neighbouring countries.

Aging is largely emigration-driven. Mortality in Lithuania is relatively high (see below) but the large emigration among adults aged 25-64 years largely explains demographic imbalances. Since 1990, 22% of the population (of 1990) has emigrated. The yearly emigration rate accelerated from 7% of the population in 1990-2000 to above 12% during the 2000s. The average net emigration rate decreased after 2010, but continues to be one of the highest in Europe, with majority of emigrants being female, young, and well educated (Arslan et al., 2014). In fact, population outflows were on the rise again between 2014-2016 (Statistics Lithuania, 2017; OECD, 2017c).

Figure 1.3. Lithuania's working age population will decline rapidly in the next 35 years

Working-age population projections - Lithuania and EU28 countries, 2014-2050, main scenario

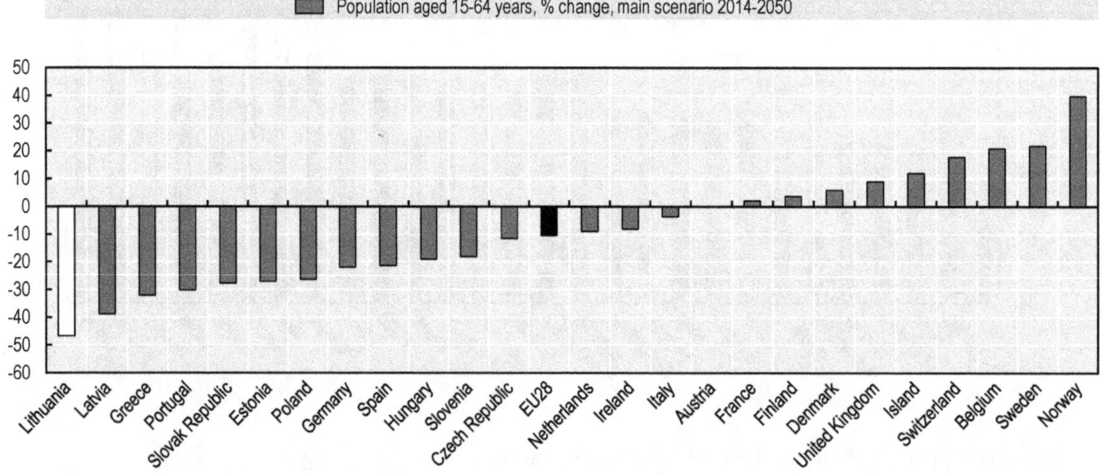

Source: Eurostat Population and Social Conditions Database; Statistics Lithuania.

The demographic change has been uneven across the country. In conjunction with these trends, a very rapid urbanisation has taken place. Four municipalities, including the 3 largest cities, have seen their population increase since 2001 (Figure 1.4). The rest have seen decreases, some very dramatic (five rural municipalities have lost more than 30% of their population). Overall these trends will give rise to numerous challenges, for instance, the need to ensure access to health services for aging and possibly scattered segments of the population. The estimates may, however, need to be revised due to the unknown intended duration of the emigration.

Figure 1.4. The population has declined by more than 20% since 2000 in 70% of municipalities

Percentage change in the population of Lithuania municipalities between 2001 and 2016

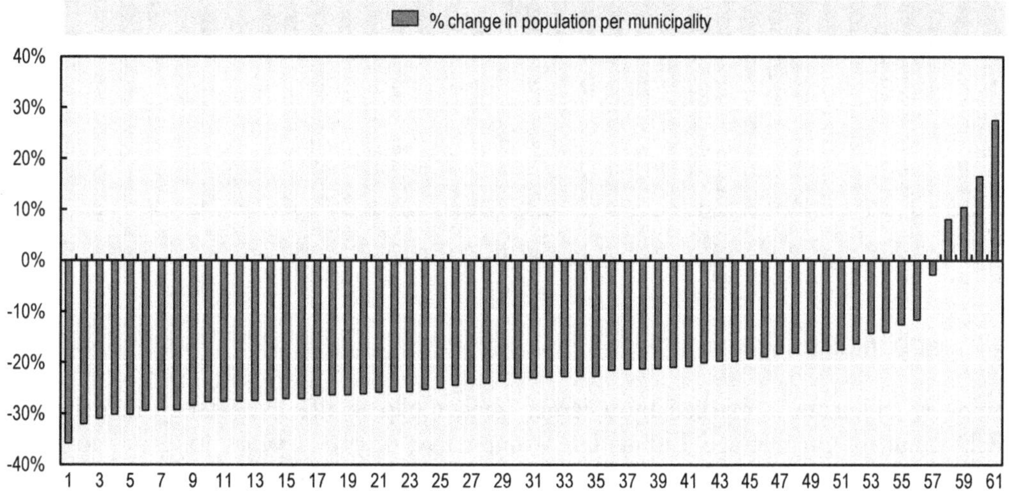

Source: Data provided by Ministry of Health, Lithuania.

1.2. Lithuania's health results put it among the lowest ranked in the OECD

This section assesses data on the mortality (1.2.1) and morbidity (1.2.2) of the population as well as the prevalence of risk factors (1.2.3). It concludes with a discussion of avoidable mortality (1.2.4).

1.2.1. Life expectancy in Lithuania remains below that of most OECD countries

Life expectancy is lower than anywhere in the OECD

Life expectancy at birth is six years below the OECD average. It lags approximately nine years below the life expectancy in the top three OECD countries – Japan, Spain, and Switzerland (Figure 1.5). It is also relatively low when compared to Estonia and most Central European Countries. Furthermore, over the past 45 years, Lithuania's accumulated gain in average life expectancy at birth has been less than four years. This is lower than in the OECD, where on average the life expectancy has increased by 10.5 years between 1970 and 2015. This trend however is typical of many post-Soviet countries which experienced large increases in mortality rates in the period around the break-up of the Soviet Union. Indeed, in Lithuania life expectancy dropped by 4 years between 1986 and 1993 and only started rising again in 1994 as the economic situation of the country improved.

Figure 1.5. In 45 years, life expectancy at birth has increased by four years only and is now lower than anywhere in the OECD

Life expectancy at birth – OECD countries and Lithuania, 1970 and 2015 (or latest available year)

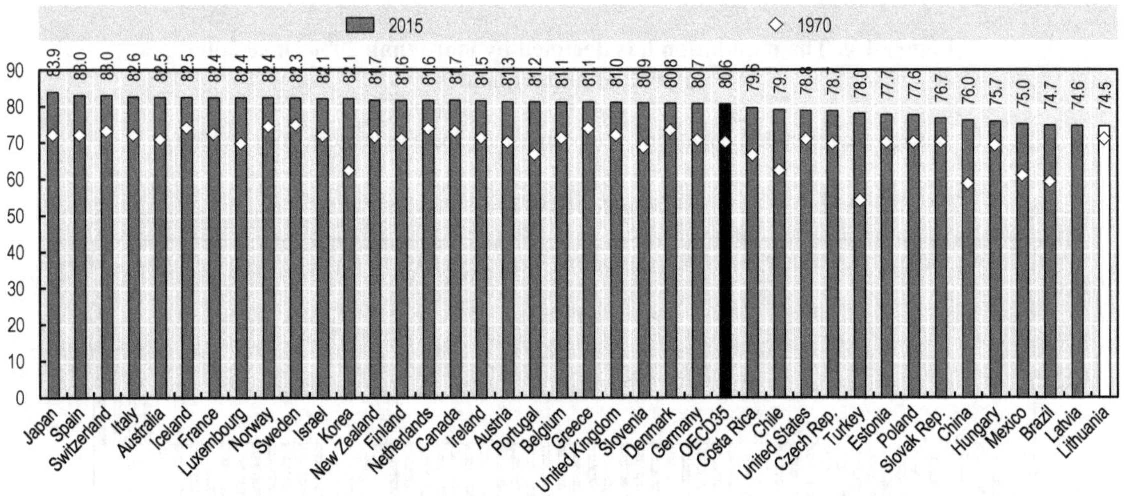

Source: OECD Health Statistics 2017, http://dx.doi.org/10.1787/health-data-en.

Moreover, Lithuania is marked by a larger gender gap in life expectancy than in any OECD country. On average Lithuanian women live nearly 11 years longer than men, whose life expectancy is 69.2 years, the lowest in the OECD. The gender gap in Lithuania is twice as high as the average in the OECD countries at 5.2 years in 2015 (OECD Health Statistics, 2017).

Chronic conditions and external causes contribute most to the life expectancy gap between Lithuania and OECD countries

Chronic conditions account for majority of deaths in Lithuania, followed by external causes (accidents and intentional self-harm). Cardiovascular diseases (CVDs - including ischemic heart disease, stroke and other diseases of circulatory system) are the leading cause of death in Lithuania, accounting for 56% of deaths (ischemic heart diseases and stroke account for 37% and 14% of all deaths, respectively) (Figure 1.6) The second leading cause of mortality is cancer – 20% of deaths. Accidents and intentional self-harm (suicides) – the external causes of mortality – account for 8% of deaths (suicides account for 2% of deaths). Death rates from external causes, which are much higher among men than women, explain a large part of the gender gap in mortality (OECD Health Statistics, 2017).

Figure 1.6. Cardiovascular diseases are the main cause of death in Lithuania, followed by cancer

Main causes of mortality in Lithuania, 2015 (total number of deaths)

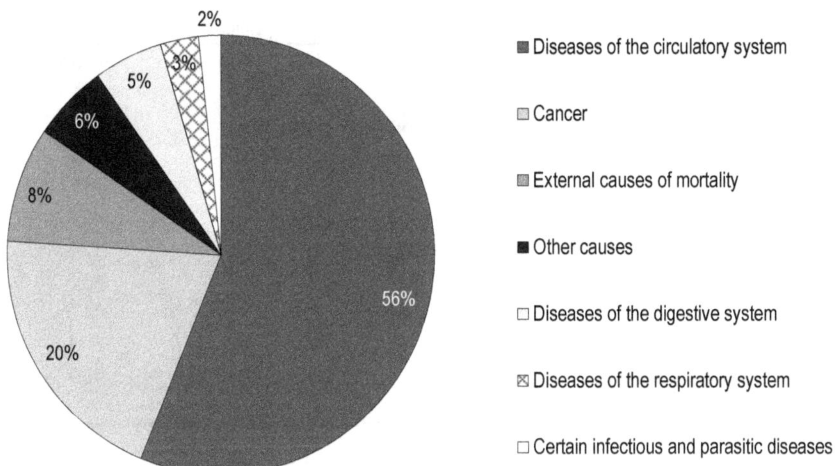

Source: OECD Health Statistics 2017, http://dx.doi.org/10.1787/health-data-en (extracted from WHO).

Lithuanians die three times more frequently of heart attacks than citizens of the OECD on average, but rates of strokes and suicides are also much higher. CVDs are the main cause of death in OECD countries, but the standardised death rates (SDR) in Lithuania are double those of the OECD (Table 1.1). SDR for ischemic heart diseases are in fact more than three times higher. While deaths from cancer occur only marginally more often than in the OECD – only 8.4% above the OECD average – deaths from external causes, occur twice as often in Lithuania as in the OECD. In fact, the SDR for suicide is the highest in the entire region of Eastern Europe and central Asia. SDR from diseases of digestive system, the fourth leading cause of death in Lithuania, is one and a half times the OECD average, with SDR due to chronic liver disease and cirrhosis nearly double. SDR from infectious and parasitic diseases exceed the OECD average by 46%, with tuberculosis explaining much of the difference. Among the main causes of death, Lithuania only has a lower than OECD average mortality for diseases of the respiratory system.

Table 1.1. Standardised death rates for cardiovascular diseases and external causes are exceedingly high

Differences in standardised death rates – main causes of death – Lithuania and OECD average, (SDR per 100 000 population), 2014.

SDR per 100 000 population	Lithuania	OECD average
All causes	1148.0	815.1
Diseases of circulatory system:	644.4	301.1
Ischemic heart diseases	422.7	125.2
Cerebrovascular disease	156.7	70.3
Cancer	228.5	211.3
External causes:	97.3	48.3
Intentional self-harm	27.1	12.4
Diseases of digestive system:	59.8	35.4
Chronic liver disease and cirrhosis	23.3	11.8
Diseases of respiratory system	33.3	64.1
Certain infectious and parasitic diseases:	19.3	13.2
Tuberculosis	6.5	1.3

Note: Raw mortality data from the WHO Mortality Database have been age-standardised to the 2010 OECD population, including for Lithuania.
Source: OECD Health Statistics 2017, http://dx.doi.org/10.1787/health-data-en (extracted from WHO).

The progress in reducing mortality from CVDs has been slow and inequalities between rural and urban populations prevail in Lithuania. The decrease in death rates from CVDs has been relatively slow by OECD standards, in comparison with other Baltic States, as well as Central European countries (Figure 1.7). In particular, for ischemic heart disease Lithuania records by far the highest mortality both among men as well as women. Regarding cerebrovascular disease (stroke), only Latvia registers higher SDR than Lithuania. While the gender gap in mortality from diseases of circulatory system is large in Lithuania, its relative magnitude is not different from the majority of the OECD countries. Geographical disparities in mortality have been decreasing since 2005 between rural and urban areas in Lithuania. Yet, in 2016 mortality from CVDs was on average 30% higher in rural areas as compared with cities (Statistics Lithuania, 2017).

Figure 1.7. Lithuania's mortality due to cardiovascular diseases has declined more slowly than in eastern and central Europe

Trends in mortality from cardiovascular diseases – Lithuania and selected OECD countries, 2014 (or the latest available year)

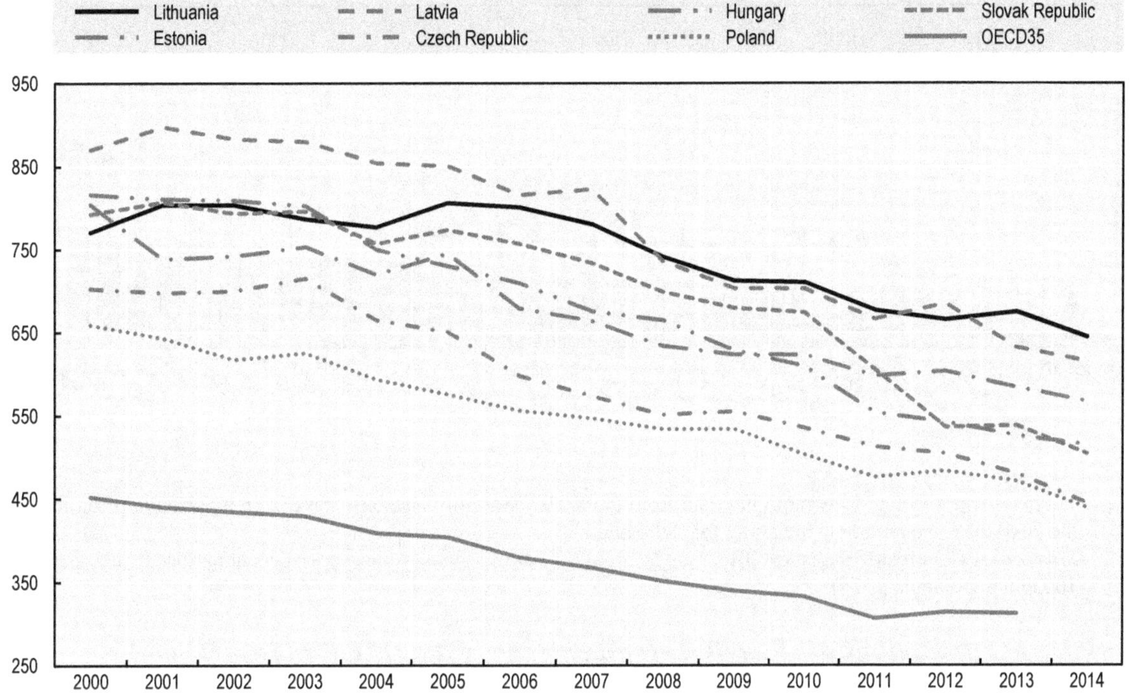

Note: Raw mortality data from the WHO Mortality Database have been age-standardised to the 2010 OECD population

Source: OECD Health Statistics 2017, http://dx.doi.org/10.1787/health-data-en (extracted from WHO).

Progress has been achieved in reducing mortality from suicide but it remains a significant cause of death in Lithuania, especially among men. Lithuania records the highest rate of mortality from suicide in the OECD, and the entire Eastern Europe and Central Asia region with the mortality rates for men being more than five times higher than for women (Figure 1.8). The problem can be partially the result of the country's history, including the transgenerational Soviet trauma - due to genocide, oppression, forced collectivisation and atheisation during Soviet times - and psychosocial strain following the rapid economic and social changes after 1990 (communication from the Ministry of Health, 2016). However, suicide rates are significantly lower in other Baltic states, which share much of the same history. Between 1995 and 2015 mortality rates from suicide decreased by 42% but they continue to be more than double the OECD average for the general population and nearly three-times the OECD average for men (OECD Health Statistics, 2017).

Figure 1.8. Suicide remains a significant cause of death, especially among men in Lithuania

Mortality by suicide (standardised death rates), Lithuania and OECD countries, 2015 (or latest available year)

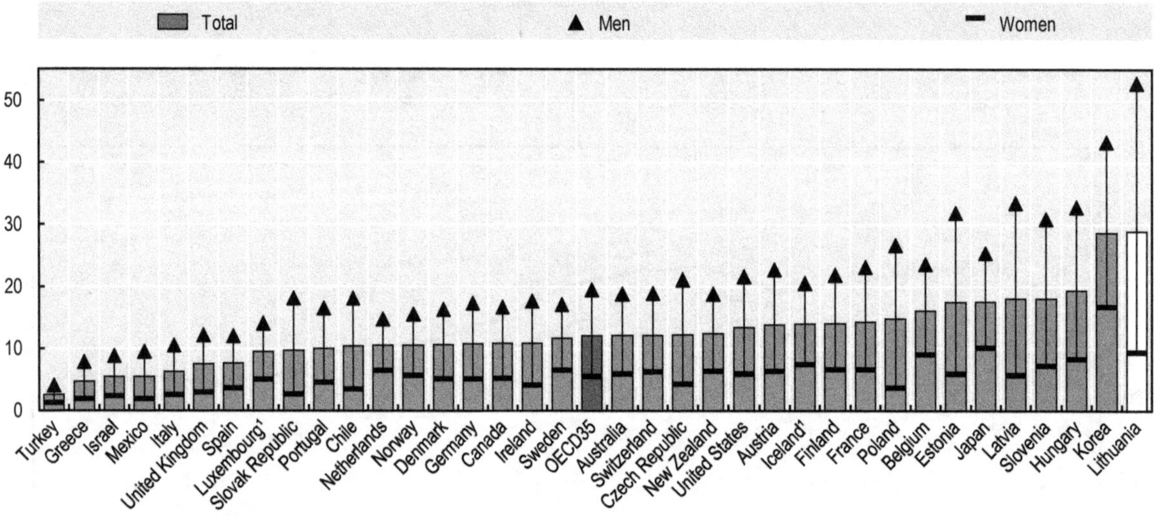

1. Three-year average. Raw mortality data from the WHO Mortality Database have been age-standardised to the 2010 OECD population, including for Lithuania.

Source: OECD Health Statistics 2017, http://dx.doi.org/10.1787/health-data-en (Age-standardised rates per 100 000 population, 2015).

1.2.2. Lithuanians are less likely than citizens of the OECD to report good health

Fewer Lithuanians report being in good or excellent health than in the OECD on average. Only 43% of the population aged 15 years and above reports good or very good health while the OECD average is 68% (Figure 1.9). The share of adult population reporting to be in good or very good health is lower only in Japan and Korea – 35% and 32%, respectively. Along with the Portuguese and Koreans, Lithuanians also most often report being in bad or very bad health - 18% of the population aged 15 years and above.

Moreover, there are large disparities in self-reported health across different socio-economic groups in Lithuania. In 2015, only 32% of Lithuanians with the lowest income (in the lowest income quintile) reported to be in good or very good health while, the proportion among the population in the highest income quintile was nearly double - 63%. On average across the OECD countries, around 80% of people with the highest income and 60% of people with the lowest income report being in good or very good health, so Lithuanians are consistently less likely to report good health (OECD Health Statistics, 2017; OECD, 2017c).

Figure 1.9. Only 43% of Lithuanians report being in good or very good health

Self-reported health status – Lithuania and OECD countries, 2015 (or the latest available year)

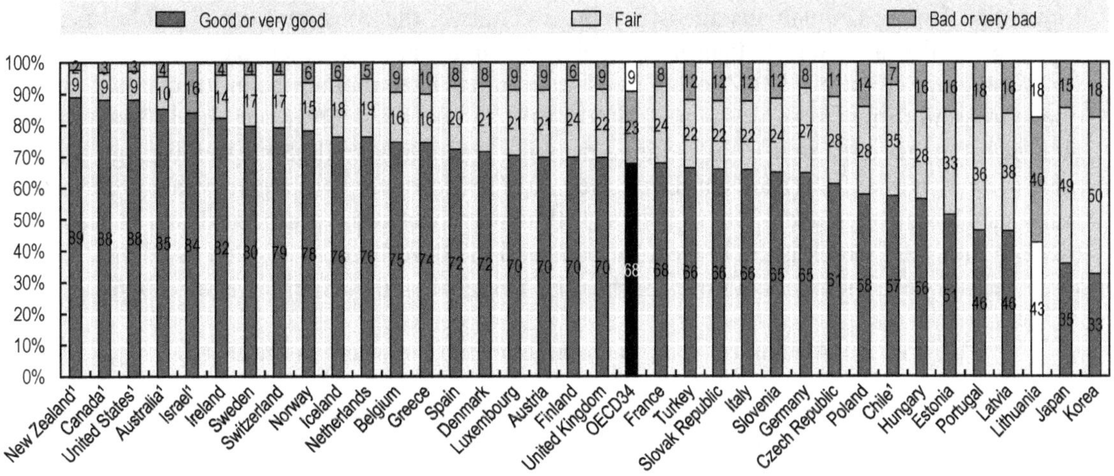

Source: OECD Health Statistics 2017, http://dx.doi.org/10.1787/health-data-en (EU-SILC for European countries)

Moving to specific diseases, data on the burden of diseases largely mirror mortality data. The main contributions to the burden of disease, as measured by disability-adjusted life years (DALYs)[1], are cardiovascular diseases followed by lung cancer, musculoskeletal problems (including low back and neck pain), and mental health problems including major depressive disorders (IHME, 2016; OECD, 2017d). Approximately one third of adults in Lithuania report living with chronic condition (a long-standing illness or health problem lasting or expected to last more than six months), which corresponds to the EU average (Eurostat database, 2017). Regarding communicable diseases, tuberculosis remains more of a concern in Lithuania than the European member countries of the OECD. Despite a substantial decrease in tuberculosis cases from 1 904 in 2011 to 1 507 in 2015, the country still reports the second highest notification rate (new and relapse cases) of tuberculosis in the EU (after Romania) with 52 cases per 100 000 population in 2015, compared to the EU average of 12 cases. An additional challenge is drug resistant tuberculosis (OECD, 2017d; ECDC/WHO Europe, 2017: ECDC, 2017).

Across the board, elderly people in Lithuania report particularly poor health. Only 6% of the population aged 65 and over reports to be in good or very good health, which the lowest rate in the OECD and markedly below the OECD average of 44% (OECD Health Statistics, 2017). Moreover, the average number of healthy life years at age 65 – an indicator of disability-free life expectancy - is among the lowest in the OECD for both women and men – 5.5 and 5 years, respectively. Indeed, more than 75% of Lithuanians aged 65 years and above report living with a long-standing illness or health problem, which is significantly above the EU28 average of 59% in 2016 (Eurostat database, 2017).

1.2.3. Harmful alcohol consumption is the leading risk factor and continues to increase

Alcohol consumption is a major risk factor behind the leading causes of death in Lithuania. Among Lithuanians aged 15 years and above, the consumption of alcohol per capita is significantly higher than in any OECD country and as much as 69% above the OECD average (Figure 1.10). Alcohol consumption has been on the rise in Lithuania – an opposite trend to that seen in the majority of OECD countries. Over one third (34%) of men in Lithuania engage in regular binge drinking[2], which is well above the average for men (28%) in the EU (Eurostat Database, 2017). Moreover, among 15-years-olds as many as 41% of boys and 33% of girls in Lithuania reported having been drunk at least twice in their life, which is the highest for boys and the third highest for girls as compared with the European member countries of the OECD in 2013-2014 (Inchley et al., 2016).

Figure 1.10. Alcohol consumption is higher than anywhere in the OECD

Alcohol consumption per capita (population aged 15 and above) – Lithuania and OECD countries, 2015 (or the latest available year)

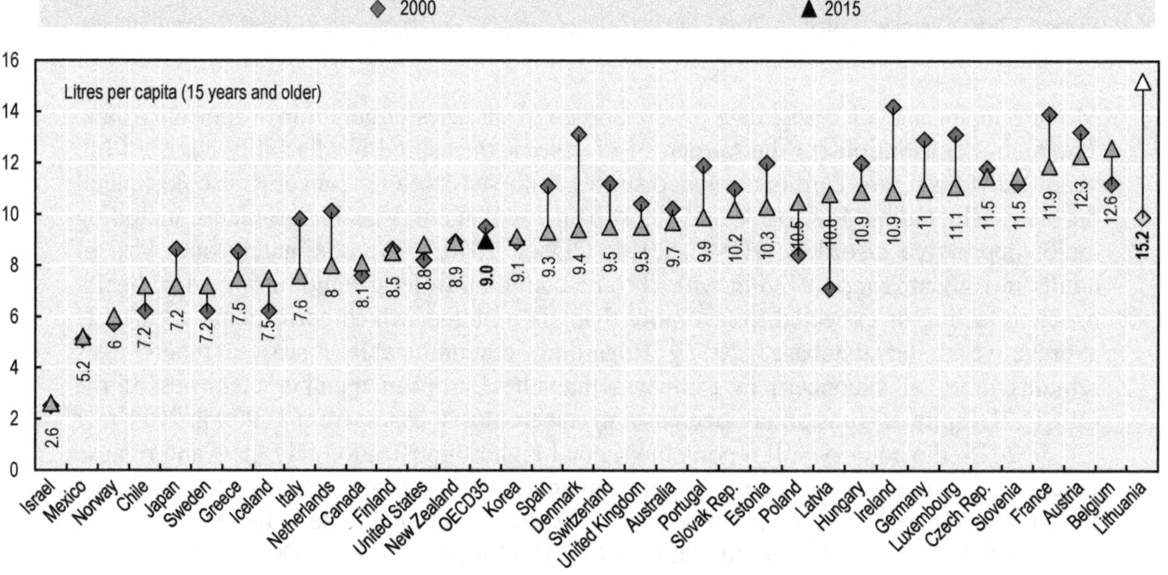

Source: OECD Health Statistics 2017, http://dx.doi.org/10.1787/health-data-en.

Other risk factors, such as tobacco smoking and obesity, are less widespread than alcohol consumption. In 2015, around 20% of Lithuanians aged 15 and over reported to be daily smokers, which is slightly above average of 18% in the OECD (Figure 1.11). This average masks significant gender differences. While only 9% of women report to smoke daily, the fourth lowest rate as compared with the OECD countries, as many as 34% of men are daily smokers in Lithuania, which ranks the country among top three in the OECD. Nevertheless, unlike alcohol consumption, regular smoking has been decreasing over the recent decade.

Figure 1.11. Men in Lithuania are among the most frequent smokers in the OECD

Tobacco smoking (share of daily smokers among adults) – Lithuania and OECD countries, 2015 (or nearest year)

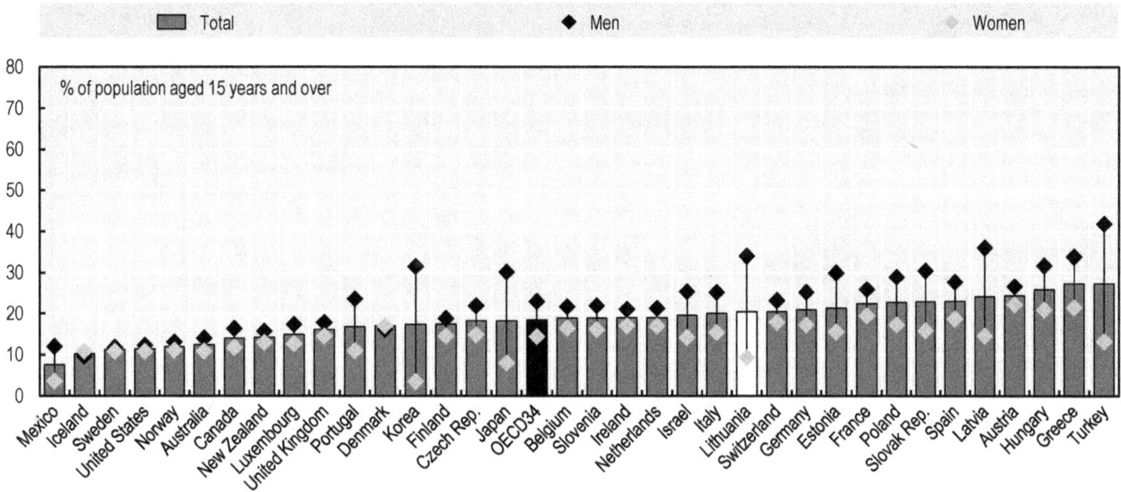

Source: OECD Health Statistics 2017, http://dx.doi.org/10.1787/health-data-en.

Obesity in Lithuania is below the OECD average. Obesity rates across different countries are assessed with the use of two different methods – either through self-reported estimates of height and weight derived from population-based health interview surveys, or measured estimates derived from health examinations. Estimates from health examinations are generally higher and more reliable than from health interviews (OECD, 2017c).Based on self-reported data, 16.6% of adults are obese in Lithuania[3], well below the OECD average of 19.4%. There are, however, significant differences between women and men in Lithuania (Figure 1.12). While Lithuanian men are among least obese in the OECD, self-reported rate of obesity among women is nearly at part with the OECD average and higher than in most countries of central and Eastern Europe.

Figure 1.12. Lithuanian men are among least obese in the OECD while obesity among women is average

Obesity among adults – Lithuania (self-reported) and OECD countries, 2015 (or latest available year)

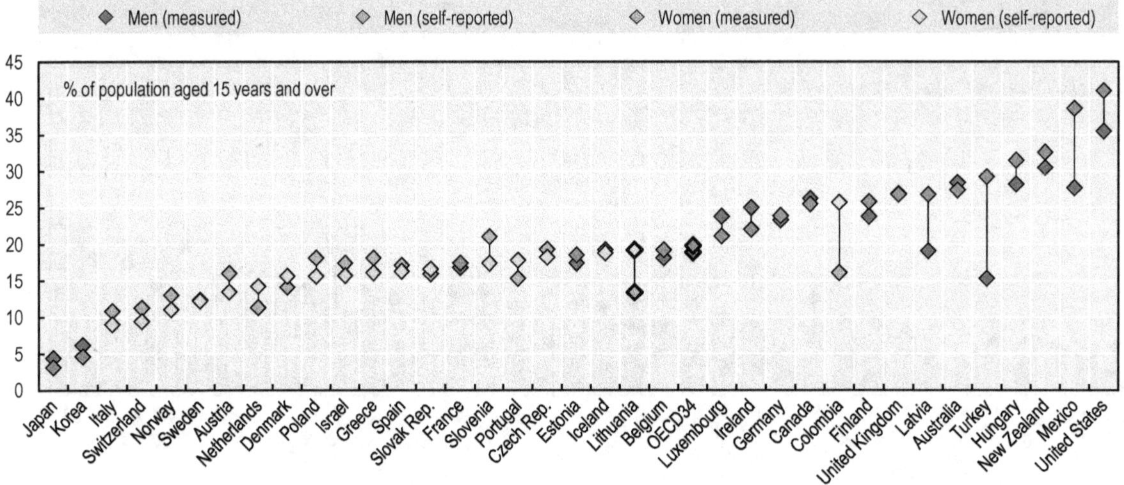

Source: OECD Health Statistics 2017, http://dx.doi.org/10.1787/health-data-en.

Overall, the gender gap in life expectancy can be attributed at least partly to the differences in risky health behaviours. The above data show that the health behaviour of Lithuanian men is markedly different from that of women, notably with regard to tobacco smoking and smoking kills nine times more males than females (Liutkute et al., 2017). Unfortunately, data on alcohol consumption is not reported separately for men and women, but the fact that death rates from the alcohol-related liver diseases are twice as high for men than women suggests gender patterns are also probably different.

1.2.4. A large number of premature deaths could be avoided

From the perspective of this performance assessment, it is important to highlight that Lithuania has among the high rates of avoidable mortality in the EU. In other words, if more effective public health and medical interventions were in place fewer people would die prematurely in Lithuania. Figure 1.13 presents two different indicators of avoidable mortality for Lithuania and European member countries of the OECD. The left panel presents amenable mortality and shows that after Latvia, Lithuania is the country in which most death could avoided through better quality care. The right panel presents the proportion of deaths which could have been avoided through better control of the wider determinants of health, such as lifestyle or environmental factors. Lithuania has the highest preventable mortality. The largest part of the amenable and preventable mortality is attributable to ischaemic heart disease.

Section 1.2.3 above discusses relatively high population's exposure to modifiable risk factors, such as alcohol consumption and tobacco smoking in Lithuania. It is difficult to separate the effect of these risk factors and other non-medical determinants of health from the quality of health care to explain the high rates of avoidable mortality. There are, however, clear indications that there is scope for improvement not only in effectiveness of public health interventions but also the effectiveness of health care services in the treatment of cardiovascular diseases. Chapter 3 of this report in particular will seek to unpack the reasons why the health system in Lithuania is not adequately tackling avoidable mortality.

Figure 1.13. Lithuania has one of the highest rates of avoidable (amenable and preventable) mortality in Europe

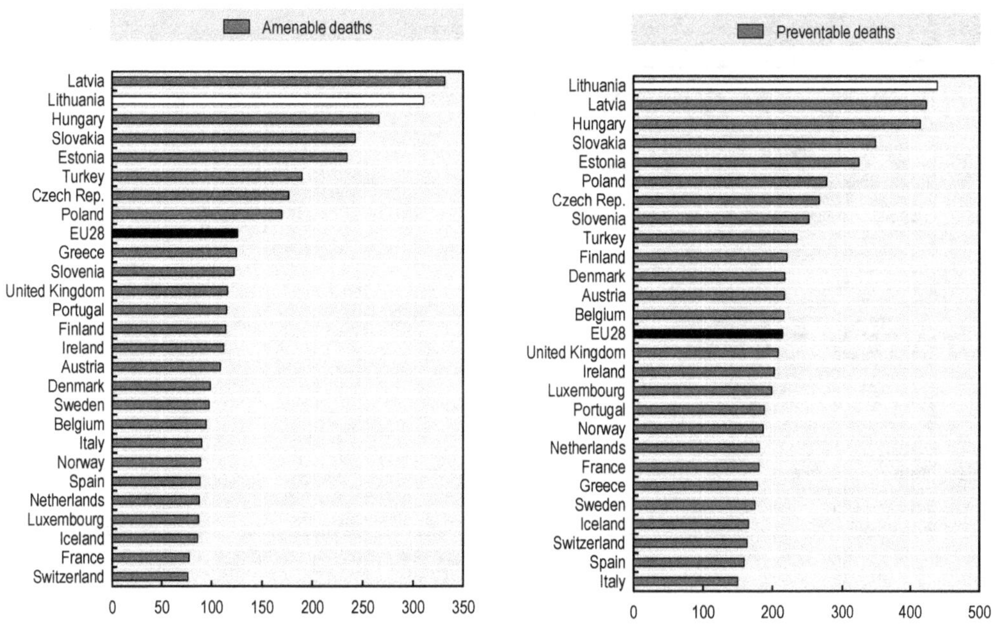

Source: Eurostat Database (standardised death rates per 100 000 population, 2014)

1.3. Health spending in Lithuania is on the low side and its structure is similar to that of OECD countries

Compared with most OECD countries, Lithuania spends little on health. Expenditure per capita stood at $1 883 adjusted for purchasing power parity in 2015. Lithuania's spending level is comparable to that of Estonia, a bit above Poland's and 30% higher than Latvia's (Figure 1.14). Spending on health represented 6.5% of GDP in 2016 (Figure 1.15). For both measures, Lithuania stands in the bottom quintile of the OECD distribution. Over time, Lithuania efforts to invest in health have increased. While in 2015, spending per capita stood at about half of the OECD average, in 2000, Lithuania's spending was only about a third of the same average. In other words, Lithuania is climbing in the distribution.

Figure 1.14. People in Lithuania spend around $1 900 a year on health

Health expenditure per capita in PPP, 2015

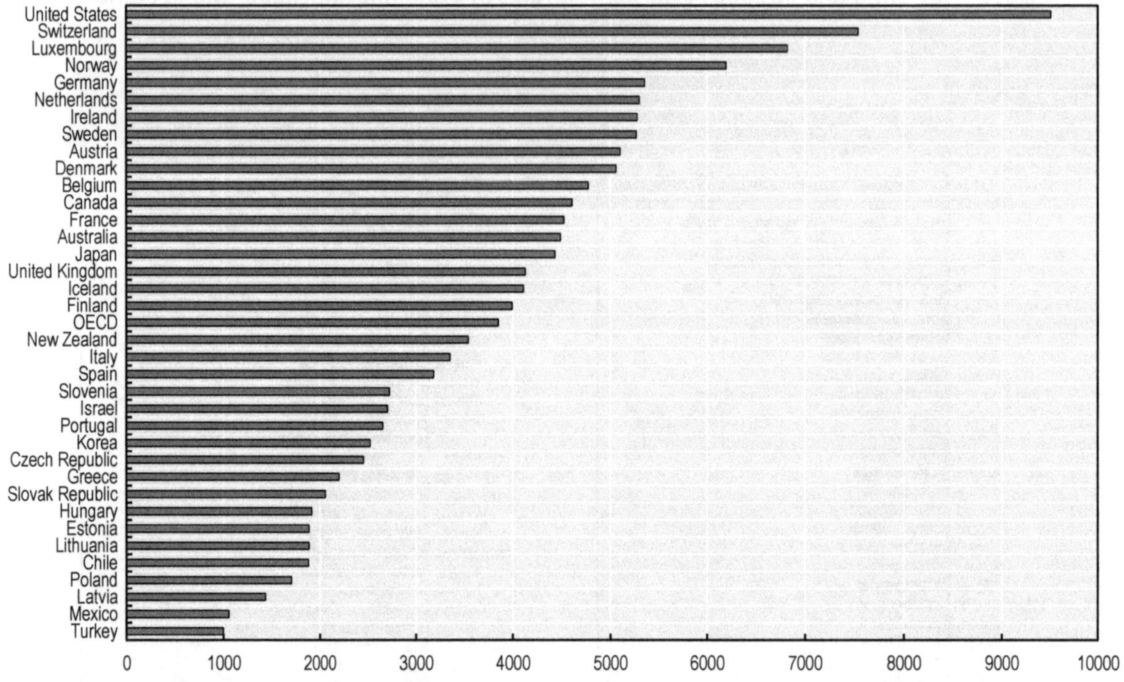

Source: OECD Health Statistics 2017, http://dx.doi.org/10.1787/health-data-en.

Figure 1.15. Lithuania spends 6.5% of GDP on health, a lower level than most OECD countries

Health expenditure as a share of GDP, 2016 or nearest year

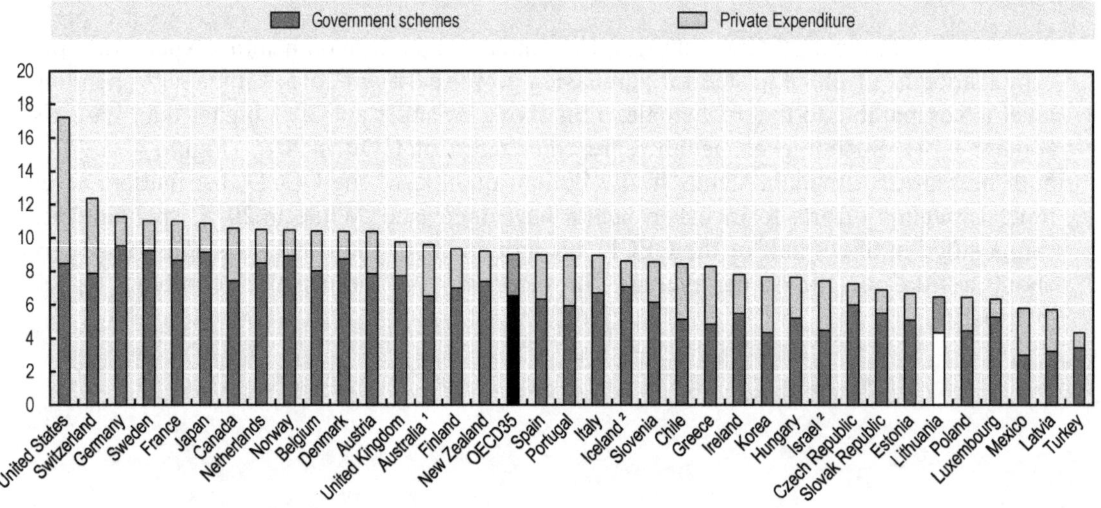

Source: OECD Health Statistics 2017, http://dx.doi.org/10.1787/health-data-en.

The 2009 crisis put a temporary break on fast-growing health expenditure. In the years leading to the 2009 crisis, health expenditure was growing much faster in Lithuania than in OECD countries: it grew by 11% annually in real terms in 2005-2008 against an average of 4% in OECD countries during the same period. In 2009, health expenditure in Lithuania reached a peak of 7.4% of GDP. It stabilised in 2009 and dropped by 6% in real term in 2010. Subsequently, and until 2013, growth in total expenditure remained slower than in OECD countries. More recently, the annual growth rate of spending has fluctuated but on average been higher than in the OECD (4% per annum vs 3% between 2013 and 2016) – see Figure 1.16.

Figure 1.16. In the past decade, spending has tended to grow faster in Lithuania than in the OECD

Growth rate of health expenditure as a share of GDP, 2005-2016

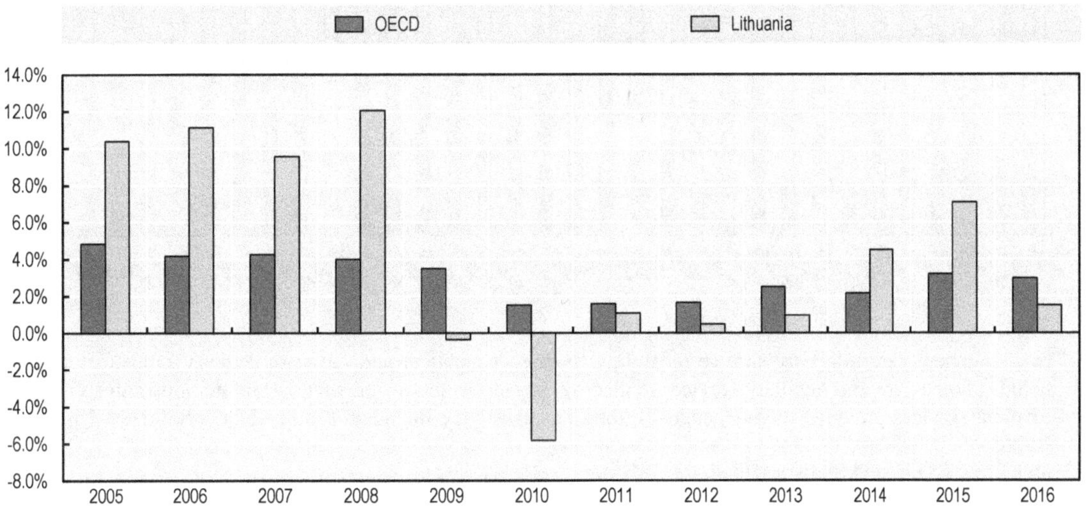

Source: OECD Health Statistics 2017, http://dx.doi.org/10.1787/health-data-en.

The majority of spending on health is publicly financed in Lithuania, but the public share has eroded since the crisis. In 2015, 67% of total spending on health was funded from government sources, lower than the 73% average across OECD countries. However, in 2015, the public share in health spending in Lithuania remained higher than in a third of OECD countries. On the other hand, public spending as a share of total spending which had been slowly increasing between 2004 to reach 72.5% has since eroded. In general, higher shares of public funding are associated with better financial protection and access for the whole population.

Figure 1.17. Lithuania spends relatively more on medical goods than most OECD countries

Current Health expenditure by function of health care, 2015 or nearest year

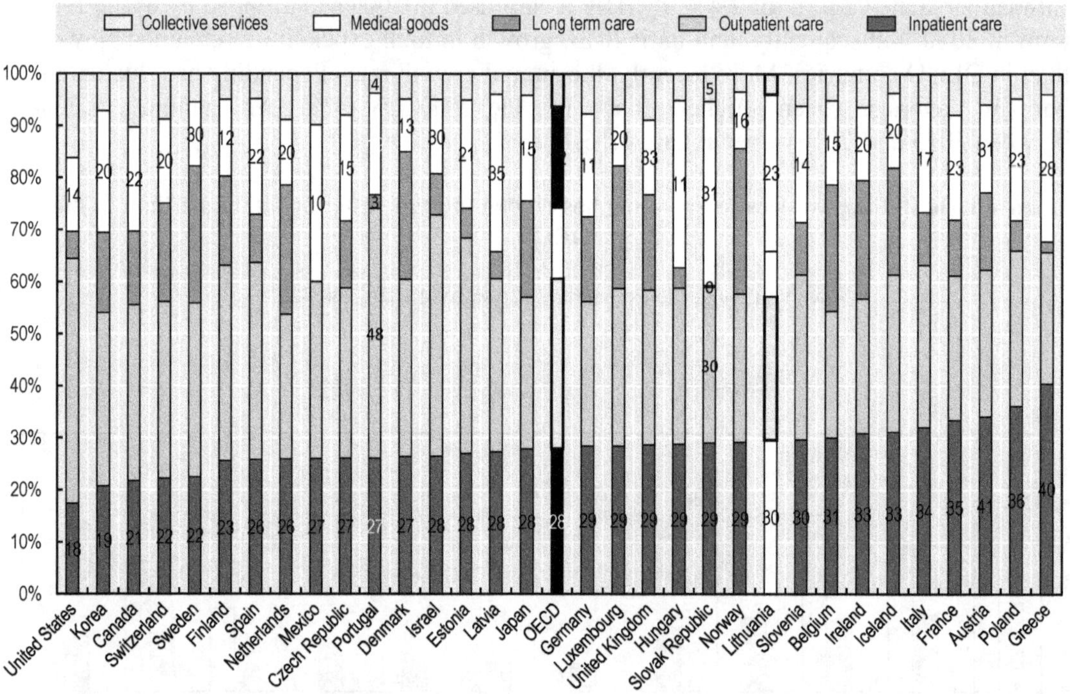

Note: Inpatient care refers to curative-rehabilitative care in inpatient and day care settings, outpatient care includes home-care and ancillary services, collective services refers to prevention and administrative costs. Inpatient services provided by independent billing physicians are included in outpatient care for the United States.

Source: OECD Health Statistics 2017, http://dx.doi.org/10.1787/health-data-en.

Inpatient services still account for a large share of total spending in Lithuania but the overall spending structure has been converging with OECD averages. Lithuania's health system – as those in most of eastern and central Europe – developed by putting more emphasis on hospital-centred care to the detriment of outpatient care and health promotion. This dominance of hospital-based care also translated into financial priorities, and post-independence policies have been consistently geared towards rebalancing the system. Today, Lithuania is still characterised by higher spending on inpatient care and lower spending on outpatient care than the average OECD country (Figure 1.17). However, the spending structure is much closer to the average OECD pattern than 10 years ago (Figure 1.18). Compared with the OECD average, Lithuania still allocates more to inpatient care and medical goods and less to long-term care and outpatient care, but the difference is now much lower for most categories of care.

Figure 1.18. Spending patterns across different types of services are getting closer to the OECD averages

Percentage point difference with OECD structure of spending by function, 2004 and 2015

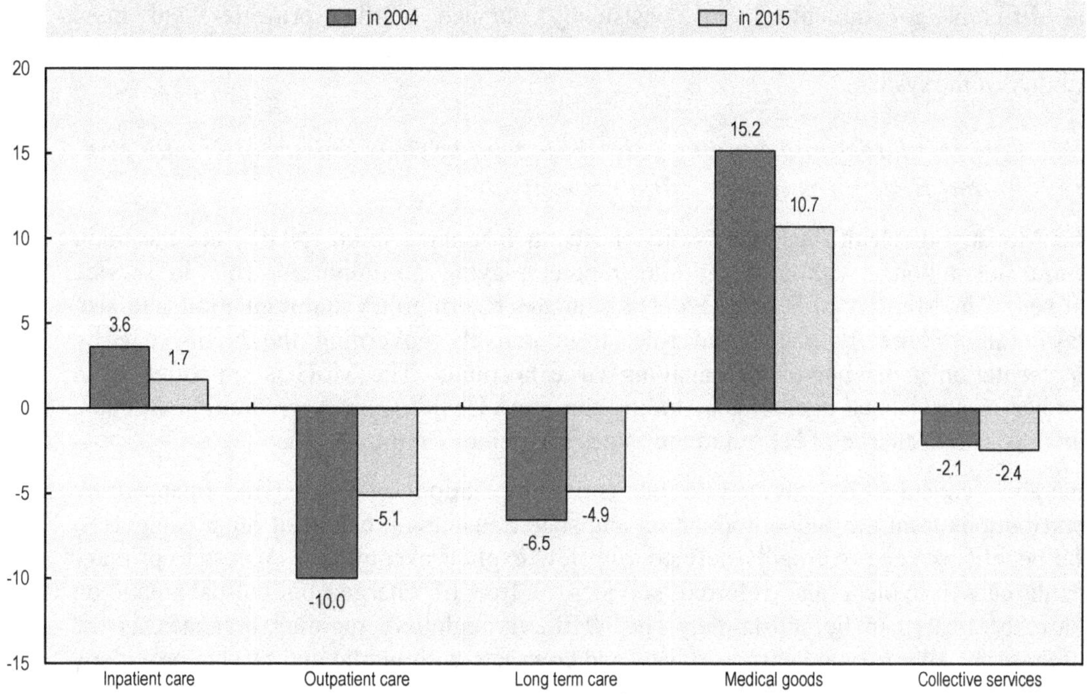

Note: In 2004, Lithuania's allocation to inpatient care was 3.6 percentage points above the OECD average, it is now only 1.7 pp higher.
Source: OECD Health Statistics 2017, http://dx.doi.org/10.1787/health-data-en.

1.4. The health system has been profoundly transformed since independence

This section describes the transformation of the system since independence (1.4.1) and presents its current governance (1.4.2). It describes the main features of service delivery (1.4.3) and human resources in the health sector (1.4.4).

1.4.1. The system was reorganised after Lithuania regained independence and has been institutionally stable since

In the decades following independence, Lithuania has achieved a profound transformation of its health system. When it declared independence in the early 1990s, Lithuania's health system was typical of the Soviet Union: an exclusively public, centrally-planned, financially integrated, hospital-centric service delivery system provided services to the entire population. In the following decade, increasing autonomy was granted to large state hospitals, and municipal management and ownership was introduced for out-patient services, local hospitals, and long-term care residential homes. The compulsory health insurance legislation in 1996 was a milestone in moving towards a contractual model with a single third-party payer and relatively autonomous providers.

Reforms in the following decade focused on reorganising service delivery by developing primary health care, restructuring of the hospital system, modernising payment systems, allocating the responsibility for public health to municipalities and introducing new regulation into the system (Murauskiene et al., 2013). With European Union accession, Lithuania made use of structural funds to upgrade its infrastructure. In the past 10 years, the different governments have consistently pursued similar priorities and most stakeholders continue to be aligned behind them, which contributes to the institutional stability of the system.

1.4.2. Key regulatory and funding role are played by the Ministry of Health and the National Health Insurance Fund respectively

The Ministry of Health and the National Health Insurance Fund (NHIF) are the main central institutions, with local administrations playing an important role in service delivery. The Ministry of Health (MoH) formulates health policy and regulation, and also plays a more directly managerial role, from actively governing the NHIF, e.g. by representation in its board, to managing large hospitals. The MoH is supported by a number of specialised agencies, including the State Health Care Accreditation Agency, which is also in charge of HTA and the States Medicines Control Agency.

Insurance coverage is provided to the entire population by the NHIF, financed by contributions from the active population and state transfers on behalf of other categories. The benefit package is broadly defined with few explicit exemptions. Access to primary health care providers and referred services is free of charge, but co-payments on pharmaceuticals can be substantial. The NHIF, through five regional branches, is the purchaser of all personal health services, and contracts with public and private providers. The 60 municipalities of Lithuania own a large share of the primary care centres, particularly the polyclinics, and small-to-medium sized hospitals. They are also responsible delivering public health activities and rely on 45 public health bureaus, which can have service agreements with more than one municipality. They are responsible for health promotion and disease prevention, population health monitoring, and planning and implementing local public health programmes. Figure 1.19 presents a simplified organogram of the current health system.

Figure 1.19. Overall organisation and governance of the health care system – simplified organogram

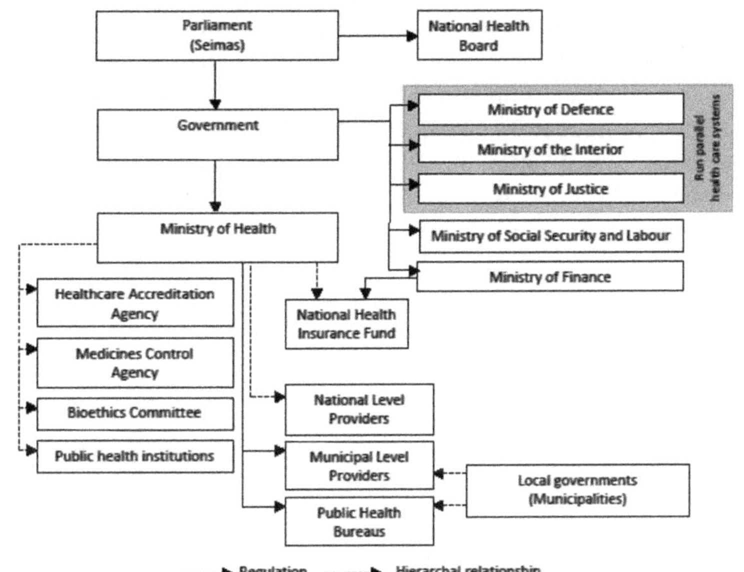

Source: Authors based on WHO and European Observatory of Health Systems and Policies (2013) *Health Systems in Transition: Lithuania Health System Review*, Vol. 15 No.2, p. 19.

1.4.3. Service delivery is mixed

Service delivery remains dominated by a large and mostly public hospitals sector but specialist outpatient service delivery is increasingly mixed. In 2015, inpatient services were provided by 70 general hospitals around the country, 22 specialised hospitals and 51 nursing and 3 rehabilitation hospitals. Private facilities play a negligible role in inpatient service delivery. Specialist outpatient care is delivered through the outpatient departments of hospitals or polyclinics, as well as by private providers. In the fast developing day care and day surgery segment, private providers, although they are still few and small, receive around 10% of the amount contracted by the NHIF annually. They also provide around half of diagnostic and interventional imaging services contracted by the NHIF.

Primary care is provided in either municipality-owned or private facilities. Most PHC facilities are owned by the municipalities. The public facilities are typically larger entities owned by municipalities. In 2015, their share of all PHC providers was 39%, enlisting 70% of the population. Private providers tend to work in small practices and covered around 30% of the population in 2015. Regardless of the legal form, all PHC providers are contracted, reimbursed and monitored the same way. Insured people are free to register with the primary care provider of their choice.

The provision of mental health care services has been considerably restructured in the past two decades, with specialised primary care providers playing an increasing role. Earlier mental health care was mostly provided in psychiatric hospitals. Since 1997, significant efforts have been made to increase the role of primary care providers in mental health. At present, more than 100 mental health centres serve as a first point of contact for majority of patients. Most centres consist of multidisciplinary teams, including psychiatrists, psychologists, mental health nurses, and social workers.

Long-term care is predominantly provided in residential care institutions but not all needs are met. Despite the fact that the national and local governments have long recognised the need to develop social services that enable elderly to receive support at home (National Strategy for Overcoming Consequences of Aging, 2004) the legacy of residential long-term services has not been overcome. This is mainly due to municipalities lacking resources and competencies to implement the services enabling care at home. Elderly in a need for long-term care frequently face no choice but to get a place in residential inpatient institutions, but capacity is insufficient. As a result, there are significant waiting times for long-term care services – in 2014, 47% of elderly in need of long-term care were on a waiting list, with an average waiting time of six months (European Commission, 2015; Poškutė and Greve, 2017).

1.4.4. Lithuania needs a more systematic strategy to monitor and address current and future human resource imbalances

Lithuania has more physicians and fewer nurses than the OECD average. Despite emigration of health staff, Lithuania has retained a high number of physicians: 4.3 per 1000 population versus 3.4 in the OECD (in Figure 1.20 axes cross at the OECD average, 2015). However, 39% of licenced physicians are more than 55 today and many will retire in the next 10 years. The number of nurses in Lithuania on the other hand is relatively low – 7.7 against the OECD average of 9.0 per 1000 population. Consequently, similar to its Baltic neighbours, the ratio of nurses to doctors is relatively low – 1.8 as compared with OECD average of 2.8 (OECD Health Statistics, 2017).

Figure 1.20. Lithuania has a fairly large medical workforce but ratio of nurses to physicians is relatively low

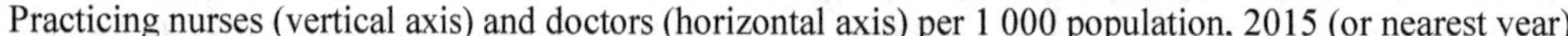

Practicing nurses (vertical axis) and doctors (horizontal axis) per 1 000 population, 2015 (or nearest year)

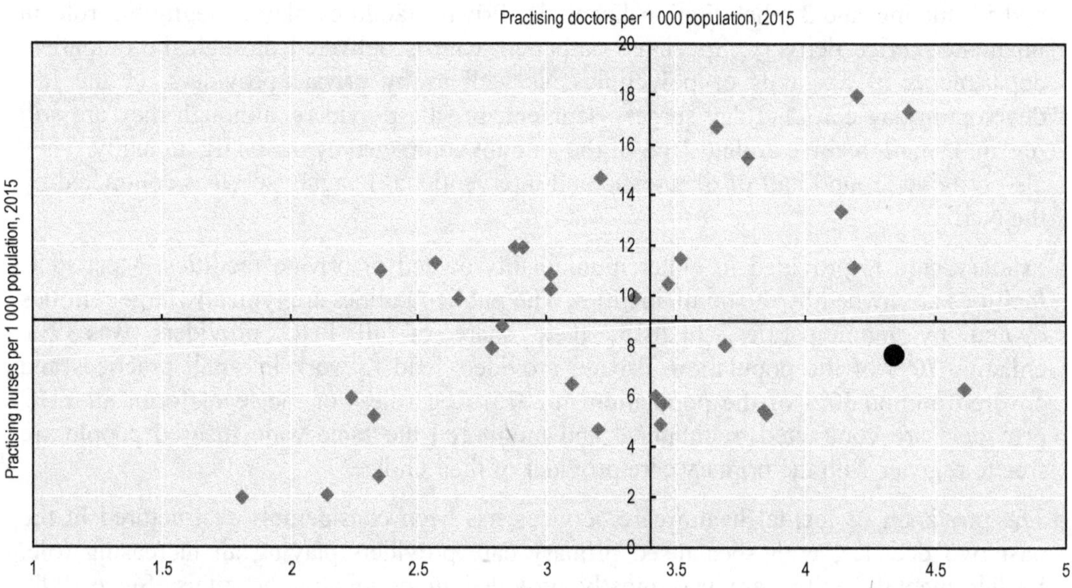

Note: Each point represents an OECD country and the axes cross at the OECD average for both dimensions. Lithuania is the black dot

Source: OECD Health Statistics 2017, http://dx.doi.org/10.1787/health-data-en.

Some measures are in place to address geographic imbalances in the distribution of staff. Specialists, in particular, are unevenly distributed across the country. In order to attract staff in peripheral areas, GPs receive a higher capitation payment for patients registered who live in rural areas or cities in which the population is below 4000, Hospitals and municipalities also offer higher salaries. In conjunction with municipalities, the government has recently put in place grants for medical students willing to work in remote areas. Overall though, no systematic tools are in place to assess future needs and gaps, or to evaluate the impact of current policies.

1.5. Improving health is a clearly stated priority for Lithuania but more attention to policy impact is required.

Health is priority in Lithuania (1.5.1) but more emphasis needs to be put on using data and evidence for policy (1.5.2), and agenda which should be facilitated by e-health (1.5.3).

1.5.1. Lithuania recognises health outcomes are lagging and the need for a comprehensive approach to tackling its determinants

Health features as a prominent inter-sectoral priority across Lithuania's main strategic planning documents. A large number of interconnected strategies and related action plans outline the country's strategy when it comes to health. "Health for All" is one of three horizontal priorities of the country's national development strategy, "Lithuania 2030". The implementation of this "Health for All" horizontal priority is foreseen by a specific intersectoral action plan coordinated by the Ministry of Health and involving 9 other Ministries which are in turn in charge of developing – and funding - their own related action plans. Another set of inter-ministerial strategy and plans specifically focuses on drug, alcohol and tobacco control and prevention (OECD, 2015a). Overall, these documents demonstrate a clear recognition that improving health requires efforts beyond the health sector.

Stakeholders in Lithuania agree on priorities which are aligned with the burden of disease and reforms which are conducive to achieving these objectives. The Lithuanian health strategy 2014-2025, adopted in 2016 builds on an earlier vision document (Lithuania's health programme 2014) articulated around a life-course approach which emphasises the importance of tackling health determinants and reducing inequalities. The strategy specifically targets the excessive burden of cardio-vascular diseases and recognises the need for additional emphasis on mental health. The programme of the new government, approved by the parliament in December 2016, makes a priority of tackling harmful alcohol abuse and other determinants of non-communicable diseases. It also intends to pursue and deepen the rebalancing of service delivery including the strengthening of primary care and the restructuring of the hospital sector. In the past 10 years, in a context of institutional stability, the different governments have consistently pursued similar priorities and most stakeholders continue to be aligned behind them. In other words, many conditions are met for Lithuania's health system to deliver increasingly good results.

1.5.2. More emphasis is required on the analysis of data and evidence to support decision-making at all levels of the system.

Policy impact evaluation needs to be strengthened. At the level of the Ministry, the above mentioned strategies and concomitant action plans are further detailed in programmatic documents which present, for each domain, the activities which will be undertaken as well as the expected results. Each document typically includes a monitoring framework on which reporting is carried out at regular intervals. Overall, this is very commendable and conducive to accountability for all programmes, but a closer analysis of the monitoring framework often reveals that they focus on assessing whether actions have been implemented in the planned timeframe rather than whether they have helped achieving the intended outcomes. In other words, insufficient attention is put into evaluating the effectiveness of implemented policies, in understanding what may or may not have worked or why and what course-adjustments might be required to achieving better results faster. Various stakeholders openly recognise that the resources to analyse results and policy impact are limited. Developing in-house capacity or partnering with outside (academic) institutions, including those who collect data, are options which should be explored to design more sophisticated logical frameworks and better understand – and transparently demonstrate - policy impact.

Lithuania's already rich data infrastructure must be more systematically put to use to analyse and hold stakeholders accountable for performance. Institutions which deliver services, in particular hospitals and primary care providers, all report on numerous performance indicators to the NHIF, the Ministry of Health and related institutions (although private providers tend to under-report). In many cases, this information is made public and availed to patients in a way which allows them to access it on a facility by facility basis, which is conducive to transparent decision making. For hospitals at least, the Ministry holds an annual meeting to discuss performance with all facilities. However, the available data is often not used to its full extent or synthesised in a way which could systematically and easily be used to compare performance. Summary statistics, dashboards or league tables are not readily available, and joint-analysis of data coming from different information systems is not undertaken. Despite their important role in service provision and public health, no information is available about the relative performance of municipalities and/or local health systems. Information is also not fully exploited. For instance, although cancer registries exist, data on survival rates is not available.

Recent steps show progress in this direction. The MOH decision to report to the OECD the Health Care Quality Indicator database in 2017 is a welcome development. A December 2017 order established a list of quality and efficiency indicators used to in order to assess each hospital's performance. Still, overall, additional resources and efforts are required to facilitate data-driven performance assessment and decision making.

1.5.3. The e-health infrastructure, still under development, will also facilitate information driven decision making

Since the early 2000s, a comprehensive eHealth system has been developed. In 2017, 12 types of medical records (including prescriptions, referrals, hospital discharge summaries, outpatient visit summaries, laboratory tests, radiological image reports) and 8 certificates (birth, death etc.) can be electronically produced, stored, and exchanged. The information is linked to a unique patient Electronic Health Record (EHR) which can be accessed by providers and patients.

The reach of e-health is expanding. As of March 2018, 554 health care institutions (out of 900) were connected to the eHealth system and had sent at least one document electronically, which is more than double the number a year before (all figures provided by the Ministry of Health). An additional 121 have expressed interest in concluding a data provision agreement and join the system. Providers who are not fully connected can consult the available information through a secure portal. By the end 2017, EHRs had been created for nearly 95% of the population and more than 15 million medical documents were stored electronically (around 5 records per EHR, when the coverage one year earlier was 70% of the population and one record per EHR). However, not all patient health data is currently provided to the central system and it will take time for e-Health to be embedded in the system.

Electronic data collection has also been established for the purpose of monitoring and publicly reporting waiting times for PHC services, specialised out-patient consultations, in- patient and day-surgery, as well as selected expensive examinations (e.g. CT scanning). The waiting time data is collected by the NHIF and reported to the Ministry of Health as well as the public on monthly basis.

The eHealth system is to be completed under the current E-Health System Development Programme 2017-2025 and The Action plan of E-Health System Development Program for 2018-2025. Yet, the details on funding and organisation of the remaining infrastructure investments are not entirely clear. Past implementation strategies suffered from inconsistencies that contributed to sub-optimal use of funding and created resistance among providers. Many hospitals, for instance, invested in local e-health systems that were later made obsolete by the national infrastructure developed by the MoH. Lessons should be drawn from these examples in order to ensure a successful completion of the system by 2025. Moreover, it would be worthwhile to explore how the eHealth system could lower the providers' workload related to data reporting by, for example, being used for the purpose of activity reporting to the NHIF.

Conclusion

After the collapse of the central planning system in 1991, Lithuania experienced a difficult but rapid transition to market economy. Growth has generally been faster than in OECD countries, but the economy has been vulnerable to external shocks and still faces serious challenges such as high income inequality and a large share of a fast-aging population at risk of poverty.

Along with the economic progress, Lithuania has achieved a profound transformation of its health system in the decades following independence. Lithuania provides coverage to its population through a single health insurance scheme which contracts public and private service providers. Primary health care is well developed and the restructuring of the hospital system in progress. Modern payment methods and regulations have been steadily introduced, in a general context of institutional stability. Most institutional elements of well-performing systems are in place but health spending remains low by OECD standards and out-of-pocket payments represent a larger share than in most OECD countries.

Despite the substantial progress, Lithuania continues to face important challenges as the health status of the population ranks among poor performers of the OECD countries. While the burden of disease is not dissimilar to that of the OECD countries, most of them have achieved more rapid progress in reducing mortality rates. Behavioural health risk factors are not well controlled, especially harmful alcohol consumption which is markedly higher than in any OECD country and continues to increase.

These challenges are well recognised in Lithuania and there is a remarkable consensus among stakeholders behind priorities which are aligned with the burden of disease and reforms which are conducive to achieving these objectives. At the same time, insufficient attention is given to evaluating the effectiveness of the policies implemented and in understanding the course-adjustments required to achieving better results faster. Lithuania's already rich data infrastructure must be more systematically put to use to analyse and hold stakeholders accountable for performance. This message carries across the following two chapters of this review which examine in greater details four dimensions of performance: access and sustainability (Chapter 2), quality and efficiency (Chapter 3).

Notes

1. DALY is an indicator used to estimate the total number of years lost due to specific diseases and risk factors. One DALY equals one year of healthy life lost (IHME)

2. Binge drinking behaviour is defined as consuming six or more alcoholic drinks on a single occasion, at least once a month over the past year

3. Obesity is defined as Body Mass Index (BMI) greater than 30.

References

Arslan, C. et al. (2014), "A New Profile of Migrants in the Aftermath of the Recent Economic Crisis", *OECD Social, Employment and Migration Working Papers*, No. 160, OECD Publishing, Paris, http://dx.doi.org/10.1787/5jxt2t3nnjr5-en.

ECDC (2017), *Antimicrobial Resistance Surveillance in Europe 2015*, Annual Report of the European Antimicrobial Resistance Surveillance Network (EARS-Net).

ECDC/WHO Regional Office for Europe (2017), *Tuberculosis Surveillance and Monitoring in Europe 2017*.

European Commission (2015), Gaps in the provision of long-term care services in Lithuania, ESPN – Flash report, 2015/51.

European Commission (2015), "The 2015 Ageing Report: Economic and Budgetary Projections for the 28 EU Countries (2015-2060)", *European Economy Series*, No. 3.

Inchley, J. et al. (eds.) (2016), "Growing Up Unequal: Gender and Socioeconomic Differences in Young People's Health and Well-being", Health Behaviour in Schoolaged Children (HBSC) Study: International Report from the 2013/2014 Survey, WHO Regional Office for Europe, Copenhagen.

Liutkute, V. et al. (2017), "Burden of smoking in Lithuania: attributable mortality and years of potential life lost", *The European Journal of Public Health*, Vol. 27, No. 4, 736–741.

McDaid, D., E. Hewlett and A. Park (2017), "Understanding effective approaches to promoting mental health and preventing mental illness", *OECD Health Working Papers*, No. 97, OECD Publishing, Paris, http://dx.doi.org/10.1787/bc364fb2-en.

Murauskiene, L. (forthcoming), Moving towards universal health coverage: new evidence on financial protection in Lithuania, WHO Regional Office for Europe, Copenhagen.

Murauskiene, L. et al. (2013). Lithuania: health system review. Health Systems in Transition, Vol. 15, pp. 1-150.

OECD (2017a), *OECD Economic Outlook, Volume 2017 Issue 1*, OECD Publishing, Paris, http://dx.doi.org/10.1787/eco_outlook-v2017-1-en.

OECD (2017b), *Health at a Glance 2017: OECD Indicators*, OECD Publishing, Paris, http://dx.doi.org/10.1787/health_glance-2017-en

OECD (2017c), "Lithuania", in *International Migration Outlook 2017*, OECD Publishing, Paris, http://dx.doi.org/10.1787/migr_outlook-2017-27-en.

OECD (2016a), *OECD Economic Surveys: Lithuania 2016: Economic Assessment*, OECD Publishing, Paris, http://dx.doi.org/10.1787/eco_surveys-ltu-2016-en

OECD (2016b), *OECD Economic Outlook, Volume 2016 Issue 2*, OECD Publishing, Paris, http://dx.doi.org/10.1787/eco_outlook-v2016-2-en.

OECD (2015a), Lithuania: Fostering Open and Inclusive Policy Making, OECD Publishing, Paris, http://dx.doi.org/10.1787/9789264235762-en.

OECD (2015b), *Investing in Youth: Lithuania*, OECD Publishing, Paris, http://dx.doi.org/10.1787/9789264247611-en.

Poškutė, V. and B. Greve (2017), "Long-term care in Denmark and Lithuania – A most dissimilar case", *Social Policy & Administration*, Vol. 51, No. 4, pp. 659-675.

Statistics Lithuania (2015), Results of the Health Interview Survey of the Population of Lithuania 2014 Lietuvos statistikos departamentas, Vilnius, https://osp.stat.gov.lt/services-portlet/pub-edition-file?id=20908.

Chapter 2. Health care system in Lithuania: Access and sustainability

This second chapter addresses the sustainability of Lithuania's health system and the extent to which it is able to provide access to care. Public spending on health was protected during the financial crisis and has been generally kept in check, which, along with available expenditure projections, suggests the system is on a financially sustainable path. Despite high out-of-pocket spending, available data suggest access to services is reasonable and socio-economic differences less pronounced than in other countries. Pharmaceutical policy is a domain where Lithuania, like most countries, struggles to balance considerations of access and sustainability.

The statistical data for Israel are supplied by and under the responsibility of the relevant Israeli authorities. The use of such data by the OECD is without prejudice to the status of the Golan Heights, East Jerusalem and Israeli settlements in the West Bank under the terms of international law.

Introduction

This second chapter assesses Lithuania's health system with regards to its sustainability and ability to provide access to care. Lithuania's spending on health is low and available expenditure projections suggest the system is on a broadly sustainable path in financial terms (2.1). Furthermore, despite low public spending, access to care is reasonable (2.2). Pharmaceutical policy is a domain where Lithuania, like most countries, struggles to balance considerations of access and sustainability (2.3).

2.1. Lithuania's investment in health remains low by international standards and so far on a sustainable path.

By international standards, and given its income, Lithuania spends relatively little on health (2.1.1). Lithuania made significant efforts to protect public financing of health during the financial crisis (2.1.2) and deploys generally effective mechanisms to keep public spending in check (2.1.3). So far, the system seems to be on a financially sustainable path but consideration should be given to investments targeted at improving financial protection and increasing the effectiveness and quality of care (2.1.4).

2.1.1. Lithuania spends relatively less on health than countries of comparable income

Even accounting for the fact that Lithuania's income is at the low end of the OECD distribution, its health expenditure is low. Relative to income per capita, total and public spending on health tends to be higher in countries with higher income. Lithuania lies below the trend line, meaning that, even correcting for income, it spends less on health per capita than most OECD countries (Figure 2.1 top panel). A similar picture holds for public funding for health (bottom panel). Estonia and Latvia are also below the trend line.

Figure 2.2 shows Lithuania *vis à vis* the OECD countries on these two dimensions. The horizontal axis plots total government spending relative to GDP in OECD countries, which is 45% on average. The vertical axis shows the proportion of public spending on health. On average, OECD countries spend 15% of their public budgets on health. Thus the various data points represent OECD countries and show how they differ both in the size of government (first criteria) and in their relative prioritisation of health in public expenditure. The OECD average is represented by the point where both axes meet. Lithuania lies in the bottom left quadrant of the graph. Only a handful of OECD countries have a lower share of public spending relative to GDP than Lithuania's 35%. In addition, with around 10% of public spending dedicated to health in 2015, Lithuania is also among countries which give relatively low priority to the health sector. Only 4 OECD countries, including Latvia, spend a lower proportion of their public budgets on health.

Figure 2.1. Total and public spending on health in Lithuania are lower than can be expected

Total and Public health spending and income per capita PPP in OECD countries 2015.

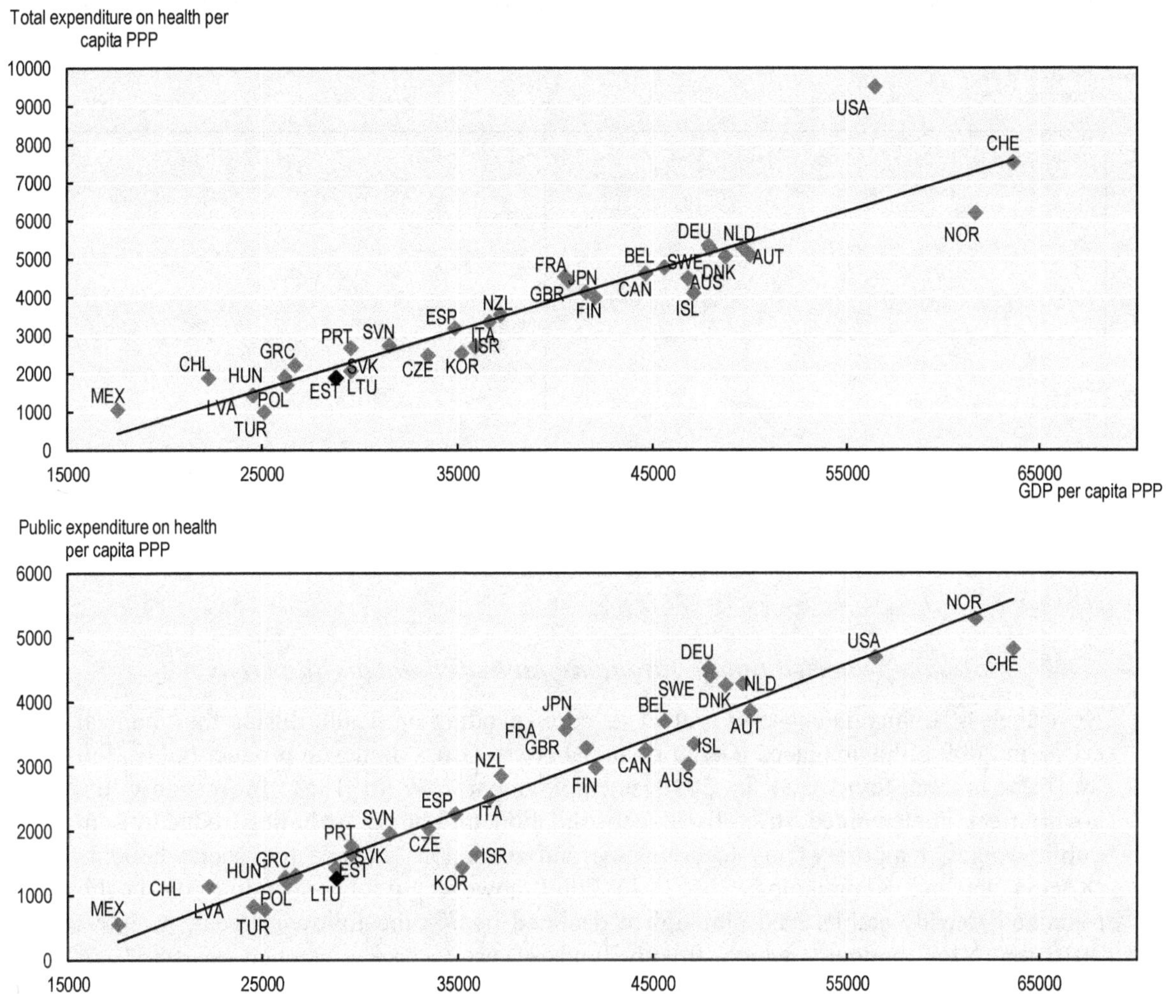

Note: Ireland and Luxembourg, where a significant proportion of GDP refers to profits exported are excluded.
Source: OECD Health Statistics 2017, http://dx.doi.org/10.1787/health-data-en, OECD (2017), *Government at a Glance 2017*, http://dx.doi.org/10.1787/gov_glance-2017-en.

Low public investment in health is the result of a relatively low level of government involvement in the economy overall, together with a low priority accorded to health.

Figure 2.2. Lithuania has a comparatively small public budget and does not make health a high priority in public spending

Total public spending as a share of GDP and share of public spending allocated to health in OECD countries 2015.

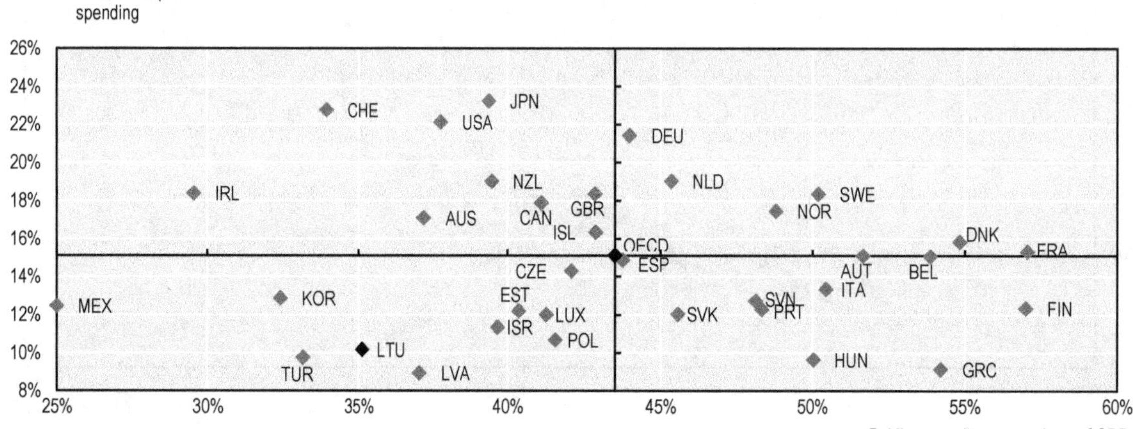

Source: OECD Health Statistics 2015, http://dx.doi.org/10.1787/health-data-en, OECD (2015), *Government at a Glance 2015*, http://dx.doi.org/10.1787/gov_glance-2015-en.

2.1.2. Lithuania protected public financing on health during the crisis

Nevertheless, Lithuania chose to protect its core spending on health during the financial crisis. In 2009 Lithuania faced a deep financial crisis. Gross domestic product (GDP) fell by 15% in real terms and in 2010 unemployment rose to 18%. In response the government implemented strict fiscal consolidation measures, including reductions in public wages, temporary cuts to pensions, and reductions in selected social benefits (Kacevičius and Karanikolos, 2015). In 2009 however, public spending on health remained roughly stable. And although it declined by 7% the following year, in 2009-2010, the NHIF budget – which directly funds access to care – reached nearly 5% of GDP, a higher share than previously (Figure 2.3, Panel A).

The mandatory state contribution to the NHIF on behalf of the economically inactive population was instrumental in protecting health spending during the crisis. The NHIF draws its revenues from two main sources: (i) a compulsory 9% earmarked contribution for employed people (who represent around 80% of the economically active population[1]) and (ii) a transfer from the state to cover the unemployed, children, pensioners, students etc. who generally are economically inactive. For each person in this second category, the NHIF receives a flat amount that is tied to the average gross monthly salary lagged by two years. During the crisis, revenues collected from the active population dropped sharply, but at the same time transfers from the state increased with the increased number of unemployed. The share of public funding in NHIF revenues rose from less than 20% before the crisis to around 35% between 2010 and 2013 (Figure 2.3, panel B). It has been decreasing again since and it stood at 27% in 2016. On the expenditure side, the NHIF reduced fees paid to most providers in 2009 and 2010, but primary health care expenditure was largely exempted from the cuts.

Overall, the public health financing architecture in place proved to be very resilient in the face of this major financial crisis and in this respect, Lithuania is widely recognised as a good practice example (Kacevičius and Karanikolos, 2015, OECD/European Observatory, 2017).

Figure 2.3. Countercyclical financing for health during the financial crisis

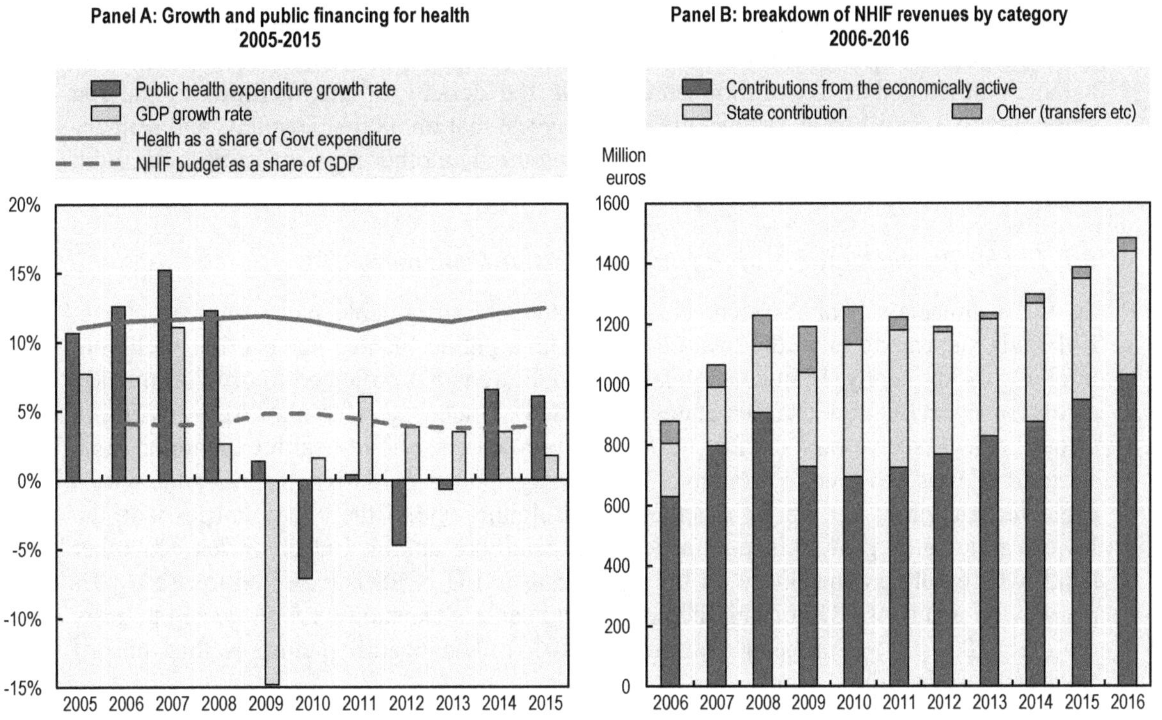

Source: OECD Health Statistics 2017, http://dx.doi.org/10.1787/health-data-en, Eurostat and NHIF.

2.1.3. Budget management procedures are effective at keeping public spending in check

In general, the laws and regulations governing the Lithuanian health sector have proven effective in maintaining public health budgets within the planned parameters.

By law, the NHIF must balance revenues and expenditure each year. Every year, a 1.5% provision is set aside from the funds earmarked to cover health care in the NHIF budget before contracts are signed with providers. At the end of each year, funds are first reallocated across providers that have delivered below or above targets, then based on local negotiations any reserves are used to compensate providers where more services have been delivered than planned.

NHIF also builds up reserves which can be used for specific purposes. The NHIF is more generally allowed to build reserves up and use them in case of revenue shortages or unexpected expenditure increases. By the end of 2009, accumulated reserves represented 7% of the budget but declined to an average of 3% in the following 4 years, reaching 4% in 2014 and 2015. In 2016 and 2017, part of the NHIF's reserves were directed by Ministerial Order to cover increases in base tariffs of personal services of 5.5 and 4.1% respectively, with a recommendation that the proceeds in turn finance planned increases in the base salary of health workers (see below). At the end of 2016, the NHIF reserve had dropped again to 1% of the budget. It rose to 3% at the end of 2017. The budget voted for 2018 planned on the reserve to reach 9% again but this plan is unlikely to hold as new tariff increases will need to be accommodated.

The finances of public institutions delivering health services are also sound (in contrast to a number of countries in the region where public facilities are often in deficit and accumulate debts). In 2016, out of nearly 280 public facilities of all levels, around three quarters posted a positive financial result (84% the previous year). Their cumulative balances amounted to 23 million euros while the deficits of the facilities in the red amounted to 3.5 million euros. Detailed data suggest that municipal hospitals and primary health care centres are under more financial pressure than other types of institutions, with larger hospitals mainly running surpluses.

2.1.4. The system so far is on a financial sustainable path

So far, Lithuania's health system is on a financially sustainable path. As seen above, Lithuania's spending is on the low side and from a public finance perspective, well kept in check. Additionally, Lithuania's health expenditure is not projected to grow as quickly as that of other EU new member states (EU-NMS). Under the reference (Aging Working Group, AWG) scenario of the 2013-2060 EU projections, public health expenditure as a share of GDP is expected to grow by 1.1 percentage points in EU-NMS. Lithuania, with a projected growth of 0.1 p.p. is, together with Belgium, one of the two countries with the lowest anticipated growth in public health expenditure among EU countries. On other hand, where public expenditure on long term care in EU-NMS is expected to rise by 0.7 percentage points of GDP during the period, Lithuania's expenditure is projected to grow more (by 0.9 p.p.) (European Commission 2015). The overall picture is thus one of financial sustainability.

The various NHIF revenue streams are being rebalanced to accommodate demographic change. All contributions are defined in the Health Insurance Law. The contribution of the State on behalf of the economically inactive is computed as a percentage of the average employee salary lagged by two year. Figure 2.4 charts the amount of that contribution as well as the average contribution of the employed and the contribution of the self-insured over time. In 2016, the contribution for the inactive was a third of the employed contribution and 65% of the self-insured contribution. In the years preceding, the contribution for the inactive had in fact tended to grow more slowly than for the other two categories. In the absence of this contribution for the inactive (or if it erodes), the redistribution between the employed and the inactive, and thus the contribution rates for the employed, would need to be higher, especially as the population covered, mostly children and pensioners can be expected to have higher expenditure than the employed. In a context where the working population continues to decline rapidly, some measures have already been taken to rebalance revenue streams over time.

Figure 2.4. The State contribution on behalf of the economically inactive is a third of the average contribution per employed person

Average yearly contribution to the NHIF of various statutory categories of population 2010-2020

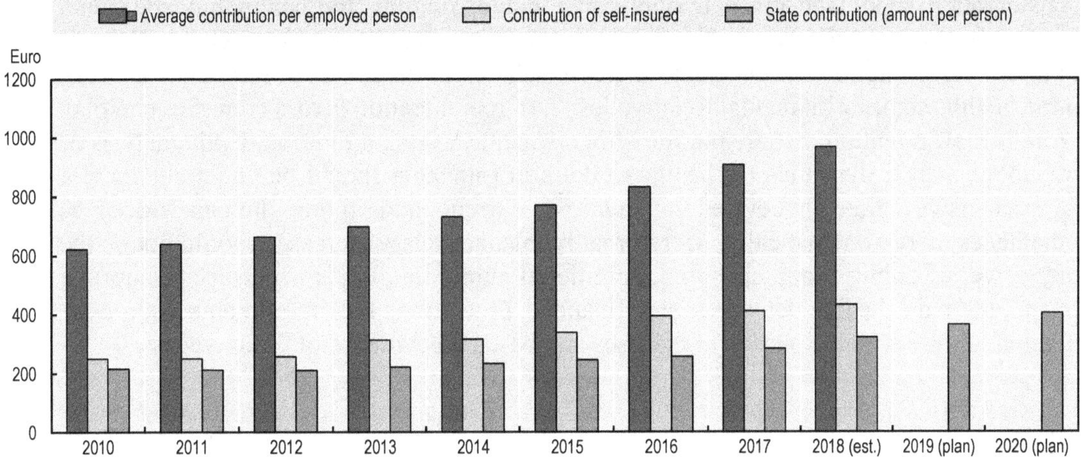

Source: NHIF. Current Euro.

Specifically, the contribution of the State on behalf of each economically inactive person is increasing. Starting in 2017, the amount per person is programmed to increase by 2 percentage points every year until it reaches the same level (in Euro) as the contribution of the self-insured, which should happen around 2021.

On the expenditure side, significant increases in salaries are being granted to health workers. As mentioned earlier, and by Ministerial order, the proceeds of the 2016 and 2017 increases in the base tariffs of health care services were used to raise salaries. As a result, in 2016, the salaries of all staff working in health institutions increased by 8% and in 2017, a further 8% increase was granted to nurses and physicians. A new agreement was reached in December 2017 between Trade Unions and the Ministry of Health to implement additional increases over the next few years. A first increase of 20% is set to take place in May 2018 for all staff working in health institutions with a priority given to those with the lowest salaries and should also be funded through increases in NHIF tariffs.

In addition, fairly ambitious targets are set for health workers salaries in relation to the average wage in the economy. The 2017 collective agreement states that by mid-2020, the salaries of physicians should be no less than 3 times the average wage in the country and that of nurses no less than 1.5 times that average. The comparison of health workers income with average wages must be undertaken with caution and differences between self-employed and salaried workers are marked, as the latter tend to be lower in most countries. In OECD countries for which data is available, salaried generalists earn around 2 times the national average and salaried specialists around 3 times the average wage (OECD, 2017). Assuming staff targeted by the above collective agreement are mostly salaried workers, and depending on how the salary target is declined between specialists and generalists, the target may be ambitious but could also align Lithuania with average practices in the OECD. As for nurses, across the OECD, those who work in hospitals tend to earn 1.15 times the average salary and the 1.5 Lithuania target may seem ambitious. In any case, statistics are not readily available on the current levels of health workers income compared with average wages in Lithuania and the cost of reaching the targets laid out in the agreement does not appear to have been estimated. It is therefore difficult to ascertain the extent to which they are realistic and whether they could be met given available public resources.

Consideration should be given to increasing public funding for health but additional investments targeted to improve the performance of the health system as whole. There is no doubt that some pressure exists to increase salaries in the hope to retain staff to work in the health sector in Lithuania. Relative levels of remuneration across countries can play a role in staff retention, but are not the only element. Overall, a more in depth analysis of the labour market dynamics for health workers in Lithuania should be undertaken and a comprehensive strategy devised to address current and future human resources imbalances more systematically. More broadly, blanket salary increases should not be the only driver of public health spending. Additional public funding is necessary to improve the population's health outcomes and financial protection, but investments should be targeted to the amenable burden of diseases and based on evidence of effectiveness.

2.2. Despite significant out-of-pocket payments, coverage provides effective access to services with limited inequalities.

Lithuania's health insurance scheme provides coverage to the population for a large range of services (2.2.1). Coverage is however not very deep and out-of-pocket payments are higher than in most OECD countries (2.2.3). Nevertheless, access to services is reasonable and fairly well distributed across income groups (2.2.3).

2.2.1. Lithuania's health insurance scheme provides coverage to the population for a large range of services

The population is adequately covered by the public health insurance scheme managed by the NHIF. All citizens and legal residents are required to seek coverage from the NHIF and the vast majority comply. As in many countries in the region, especially those with high levels of emigration, the number of residents is not known precisely, but statistics indicate that of the 3.1 million people officially eligible for public health insurance in 2016, more than 92% were covered. However, many of the 8% uninsured (around 250,000 people) are believed to have settled abroad[2]. NHIF experts estimate that the actual proportion of residents lacking coverage probably lies between 2 and 4%, many of whom operate at the fringe of the formal economy[3]. The uninsured are officially entitled to free emergency care. The state guarantees coverage for the economically inactive. During the crisis, as the number of unemployed rose, the proportion of the economically inactive in the insured population grew to a peak of 71% in 2011, and it has been steadily declining since, to about 54% in 2016.

Coverage is quite broad but patient copayments apply on most outpatient medicines. The insured are entitled to a broad range of rather loosely defined personal health services. A positive list indicates those medical goods and medicines that are reimbursed. For drugs used in ambulatory care, reimbursement rates range between 50 and 100% depending on the condition and whether the patient is a child, a pensioner, or a person with disabilities (with the majority covered at 80 or 100%). Reimbursement can also be tied to specific indications. For example, until 2016 statins were only reimbursed for secondary prevention of cardiovascular diseases. Lithuania now is aligned with many other countries' guidelines that recommend their use in primary prevention in certain patients (e.g. NICE, 2014).

The co-payment rules for medicine are complex and some recent measures have aimed at curbing them. For all medicines but the cheapest within a group of medicines with the same active substance[4] patients pay a fee of between 0.2 and 1.5 EUR per package, depending on the total price. In general, the reimbursement rate is applied to the reference price, which cannot exceed 95% of the average of the lowest prices in each of eight reference countries[5] (plus a regulated pharmacy mark-up and VAT). However, the retail price of a drug (i.e. the price at which a manufacturer offers the drug on the Lithuanian market) may bear no relation to the reference price. Indeed, retail prices of most prescription medicines are often significantly higher than their reference prices (Ministry of Health, Lithuania, 2017), with patients required to cover the difference. This markedly increases the magnitude of out of pocket costs for outpatient medicines. Since 2010, pharmacies are required to offer the cheapest generic in a group of medicines at a retail price not exceeding the reference price. Moreover, since 2017, for a brand to be included in the positive list of reimbursed drugs, the retail price cannot exceed the reference price by more than 10%. However this rule only applies to groups of medicines with at least three manufacturers (Ministry of Health, Lithuania, 2017).

2.2.2. Out-of-pocket payments are among the highest in the OECD and informal payments remain frequent.

Out-of-pocket payment are high in Lithuania, especially on medicine

In 2015, out of pocket payments represented around 32% of health spending in Lithuania, among the highest levels in the OECD (see Figure 2.5). Private health insurance is not developed in Lithuania, thus the bulk of private spending is out of pocket (OOP). The proportion of health expenditure paid OOP was around 33% in the mid-2000s, decreasing somewhat during the financial crisis due to a sharp reduction in private relative to public spending growth rates, and has risen again after 2012. Spending on medicines and medical goods represents 64% of OOP and ambulatory services another 29%.

Figure 2.5. Out-of-pocket payments are high in Lithuania

Out-of-pocket as a share of total health spending in OECD countries, 2015

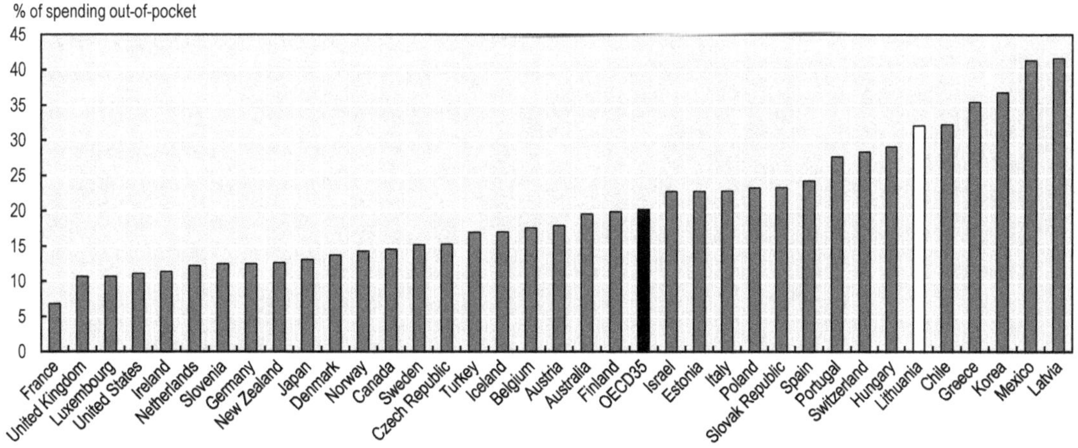

Source: OECD Health Statistics 2017, http://dx.doi.org/10.1787/health-data-en.

Coverage is particularly low for medicines in Lithuania. The proportion of the cost which patients have to pay out-of-pocket varies considerably across types of care. For inpatient care, the proportion is only 6.1%, almost equal to the OECD average. On the other hand, OOP for ambulatory care is over 40%, when the OECD average is around 27%. When it comes to medical goods, which mostly consist of medicines, the patients have to bear 68% of the cost, which is considerable (for further details on pharmaceuticals, see Section 2.3).

Out-of-pocket spending has a significant impoverishing effect on part of the population. WHO suggests that the risk of impoverishment from OOP costs becomes significant in countries where these represent more than 20% of total spending. A WHO report on Lithuania reviewed the impact of OOP on poverty (Murauskienė and Thomson, 2018). It showed that in 2012 (most recent year for which data is available) 9.4% of the population experienced financial hardship due to health spending, a reduction from the 2008 level of 11.5% but higher than in 2005 (7%). The incidence of catastrophic spending is heavily concentrated among older people (those aged 60 and over) and couples without children. Eighty percent of catastrophic spending is due to medicines, and this proportion is even higher among households belonging to the lowest income quintile.

Financial protection is a significant cause of concern, to which the government has drawn a lot of policy attention since 2016. It has been recognised that the current pharmaceuticals pricing methods is more geared towards protecting the budget of the NHIF than ensuring financial protection for patients. Several measures intended to reduce user charges on prescription medicines were implemented in 2017 and 2018 and are discussed in detail in Section 2.3. Moreover, in 2017, the VAT on prescription medicines for which the retail price exceeds 300 EUR was reduced from 21% to 5%. In 2017 the government also adopted guidelines for pharmaceutical market policy, which included a call to develop a separate model for the reimbursement of medicines for low-income patients (Ministry of Health, Lithuania, 2017).

Figure 2.6. Coverage is particularly low for outpatient care and medical goods

Panel A: Out of pocket share of spending for outpatient care in OECD countries and Lithuania, 2015

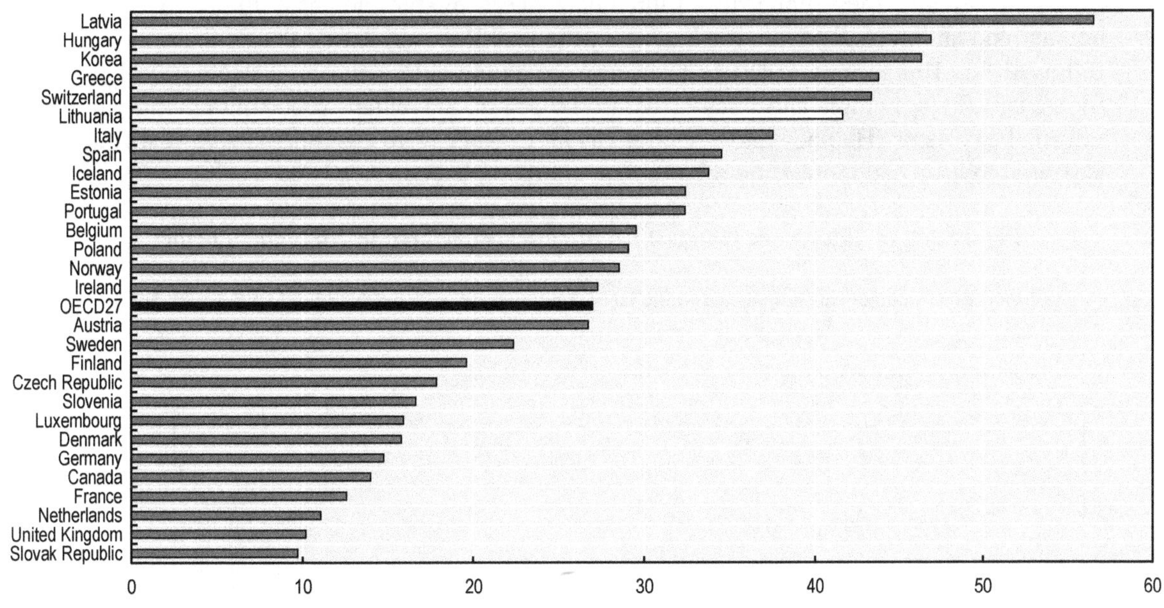

Panel B: Out of pocket share of spending for medical goods in OECD countries and Lithuania, 2015

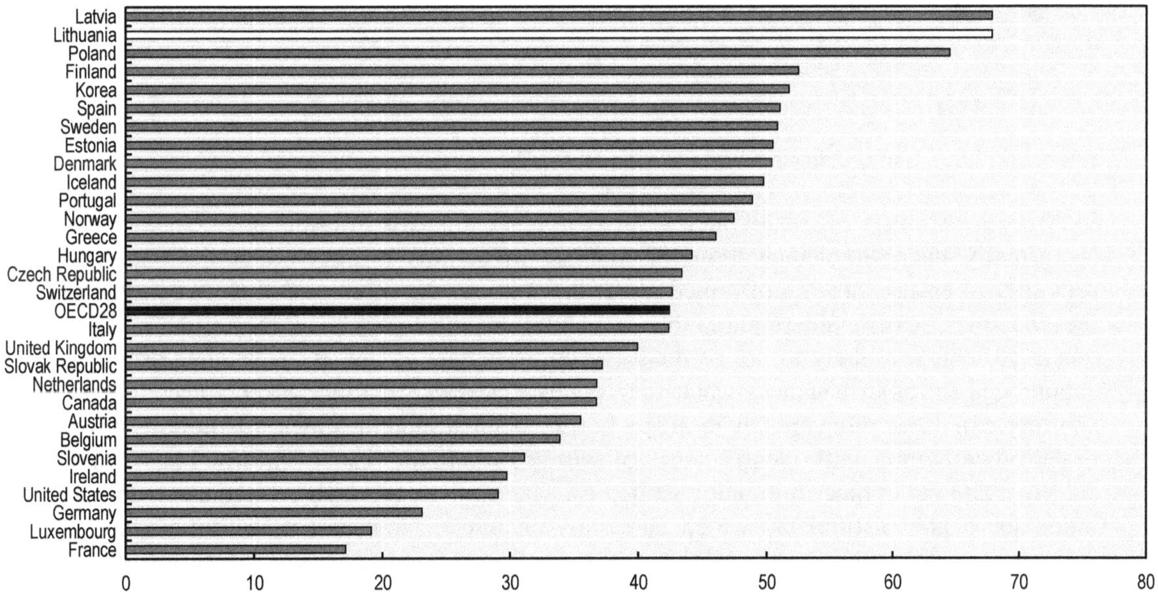

Source: OECD Health Statistics 2017, http://dx.doi.org/10.1787/health-data-en.

Informal payments were widespread in Lithuania but recent data suggest they might be declining

Informal payments seem to have been more widespread in Lithuania than in comparable countries. A 2013 Transparency International report, based on a survey implemented in a range of countries, inquired whether people had paid a bribe when accessing services. In

Lithuania, 35% declared having done so, by far the highest proportion in the OECD (Figure 2.7). These results echoed those of the 2010 Life-in-Transition survey which reported results for eight countries of Eastern Europe which are currently OECD members. Among these countries, Lithuanians were by far the most likely to report having paid an informal payment when using the health care system: 40% of them did so, followed by Hungarians (34). The rates were below 20% in the Czech Republic, Slovakia, Latvia, Estonia and Poland, with only 3% of Slovenians reporting having paid informal payments (Habibov and Cheung, 2017). In other words, Lithuania five years ago appeared to have had more of a problem than comparable countries.

Figure 2.7. In 2013, more than a third of patients declared having paid a bribe

Proportion of people who sought care in the last 12 months and paid a bribe, OECD and Lithuania

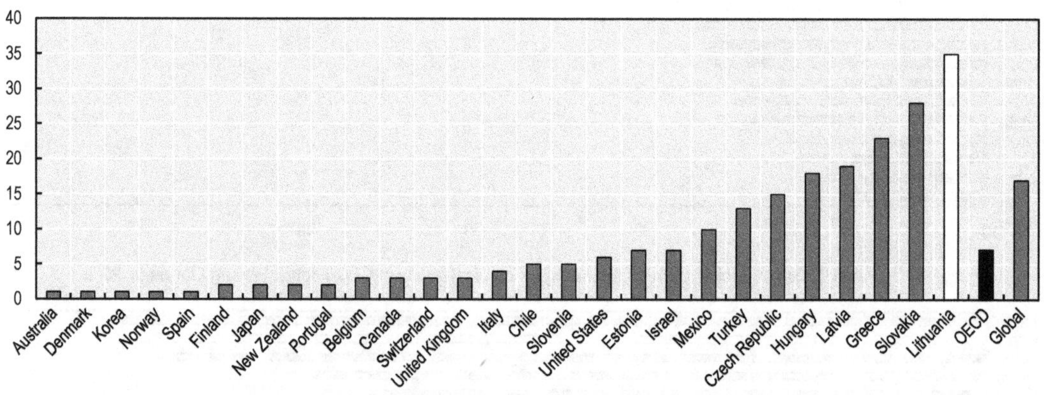

Source: TI (2013), Global Corruption Barometer Report and Data, http://www.transparency.org/gcb2013.

In 2015, the Ministry of Health put a strategy in place to tackle informal payments, which is currently under implementation. A first set of actions is directed at the patients, primarily to ensure they are informed about the services they are entitled to and possible fees they may be officially required to pay. Institutions must post this information in areas where patients are likely to notice them (reception areas, wards, etc.). Patients are also encouraged to report instances when they believe they were unduly asked for payments and they can do so anonymously though a hotline open around the clock. Institutions have to periodically train staff, identify areas of services where the risks of informal payments are high, and put in place mitigation strategies. The Ministry has also created a corruption index for health institutions, which can translate into a "transparent institution label" being granted to facilities and is also meant to be factored in to compute the performance component of salaries of key managerial staff in public institutions.

Recent data suggest that informal payments are decreasing. Indeed, in the most recent wave of the Transparency International survey published in 2016, 24% of Lithuanian reported a bribe when they used the health service in the past year (against 35% in 2013). The most recent Eurobarometer on corruption also points to a decreasing trend. In 2017, only 12% of people who had been in contact with the system in the previous year declared having made a non-official fee or gift to the doctor, nurse or hospital, when in 2013 the proportion was 21%. While these 2017 numbers are encouraging, and lower than in Romania (19%) and Hungary (17%), in 20 countries of the EU, fewer than 5% declare having made such payments (European Commission 2017).

2.2.3. By and large coverage translates into access to services for all the population

The number of contacts per population with the system are on the high side

Compared with OECD averages, people in Lithuania access health services frequently. In 2016, individuals consulted physicians on average 8.8 times a year, nearly 20% above the OECD average (Figure 2.8, Panel A). Around two thirds of these visits were to primary care physicians (NHIF data). In 2015 there was an average of 24 hospital discharges per 1000 population. This is the third highest discharge rate among OECD countries and 50% above the average (Figure 2.8, Panel B). This suggests that access to services is not constrained.

Figure 2.8. People in Lithuania access doctors and hospitals frequently

Panel A: Number of doctor consultations per person, 2000 and 2015 (or nearest year)

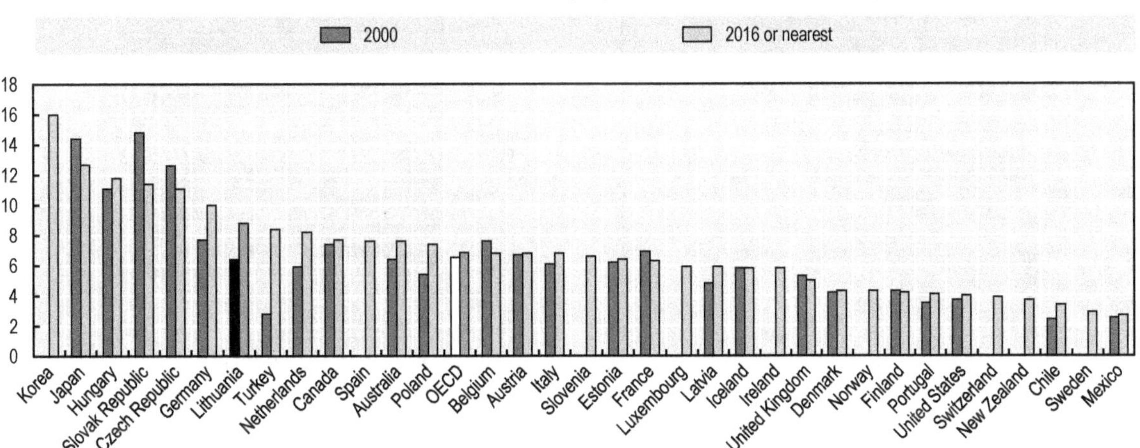

Panel B: Number of hospital discharges per 1000 person, 2000 and 2014 (or nearest year)

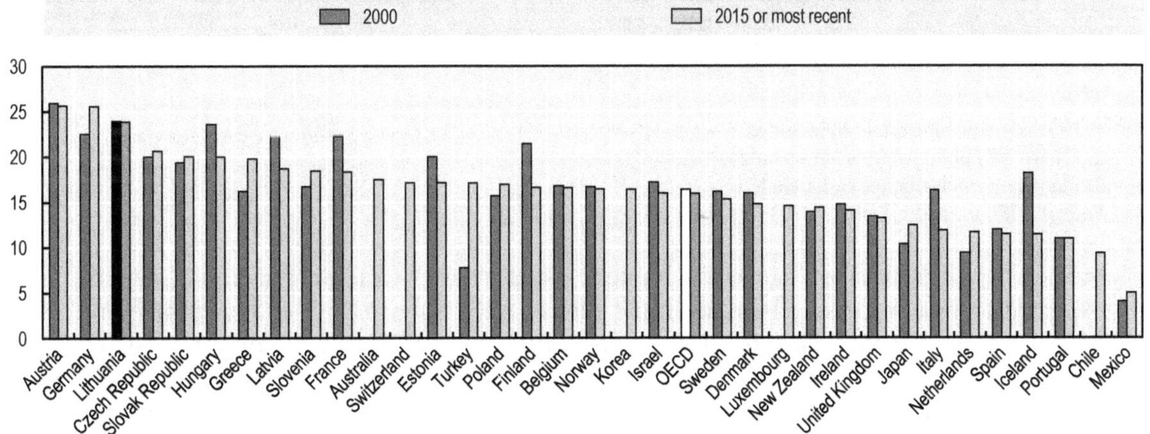

Source: OECD Health Statistics 2017, http://dx.doi.org/10.1787/health-data-en.

On the other hand, the number of diagnostic imaging tests provided to patients is below the OECD average. Figure 2.9 presents the number of tests per 1000 population in the OECD and Lithuania for MRIs (Panel A) and CT scans (Panel B). The levels are lower than in most OECD countries reporting data. The number of PET scans per 1000 population is 0.5, comparable to the number in Finland and a bit below Estonia (0.9) but much lower than the in other 15 OECD countries reporting data (3 PET scans per 1000 population). It is important however to keep in mind that when it comes to imaging tests, higher numbers do not necessarily mean better care. Medical imaging is one of the domains where often many tests are being conducted which have low value. If access is to be developed in Lithuania, every effort should be made to ensure it is embedded in best practice clinical guidelines and takes into account recommendations such as those of Choosing Wisely ®, a campaign and international movement which promotes appropriate care.

Figure 2.9. The volumes of diagnostic imaging services are on the low side

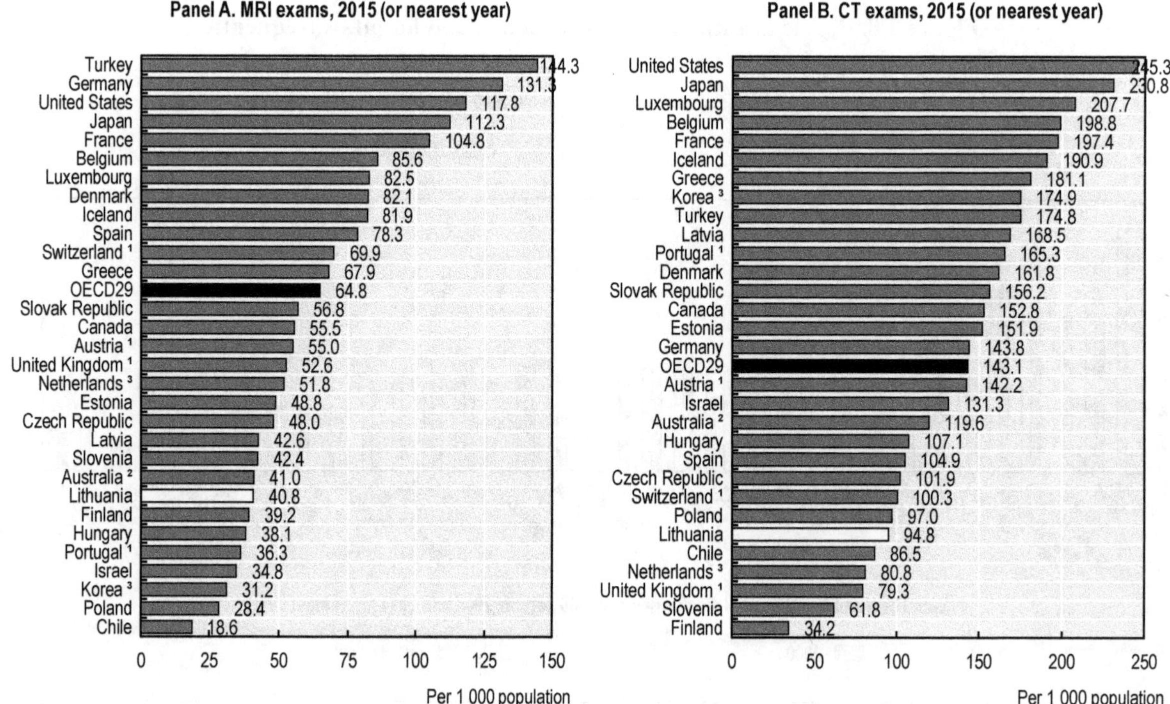

1. Exams outside hospital not included.
2. Exams on public patients not included.
3. Exams privately-funded not included.
Source: OECD Health Statistics 2017, http://dx.doi.org/10.1787/health-data-en.

Inequalities in access are currently limited, but a minority of the population can be expected to face increasing barriers in the future. According to both administrative and survey data geographical inequalities are not stark. At least 72% of the rural population declared having seen a primary care provider in the previous year, compared with 75% of the urban population (Statistics Lithuania, 2015). Figure 2.10 is based on the average number of consultations per municipality and presents the share of the population living in the municipalities with different volumes of visits per year. Across municipalities, the number of outpatient visits per capita per year ranges from 2.9 to nearly 13 (with an average of 8.7), but 93% of the population lives in municipalities where the average number of contacts with outpatient physicians exceeds 5 per year. Around half of the remaining 7% live in municipalities adjacent to large cities, which suggest that geographic barriers to access may not be insurmountable. The rest, however, live in remote municipalities and ensuring their access to services is likely to be difficult. As the population is decreasing very rapidly in some parts of Lithuania, efforts will be needed to develop innovative solutions in this regard.

Figure 2.10. The vast majority of the population lives in areas where people see a physician at least five times per year on average

Proportion of the population living in municipalities with different levels of outpatient visits per capita 2016

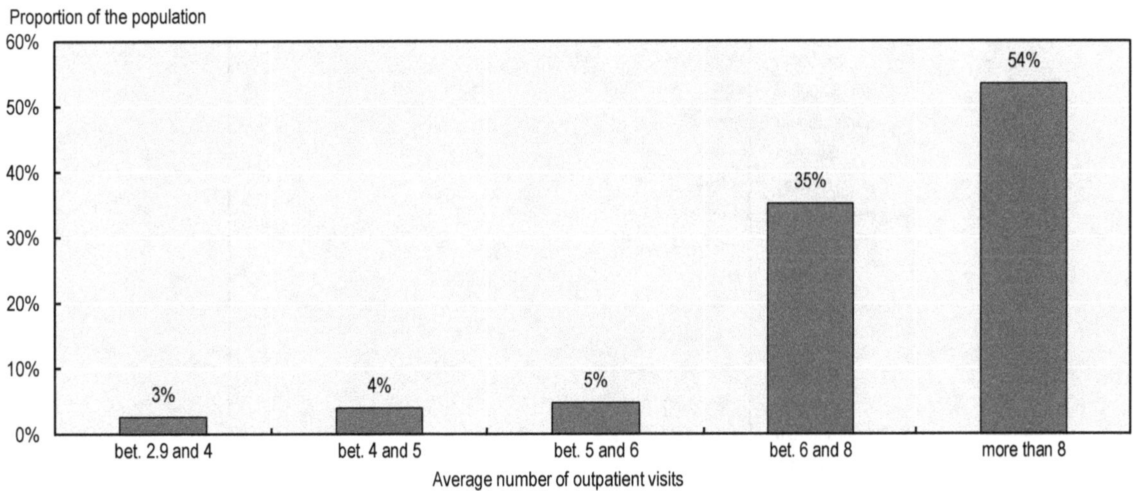

Source: NHIF data.

Unmet needs are lower than in comparable countries

Survey data also suggest barriers to access are limited. In the 25 EU countries of the OECD, on average, 3.2% of the population declared not having sought care for financial, geographic or waiting time reasons in 2015, compared with 2.9% in Lithuania. In addition, in most countries where the proportion of the population foregoing care exceeds 2%, individuals in low income households are much more likely than those in high income households to do so. In Lithuania, this difference is relatively small (Figure 2.11). Higher proportions of people foregoing care and/or wider inequalities can be found in many European countries, including Latvia and Estonia. The most recent wave of the European Health Interview Survey (EHIS), carried it out in 2014 in Lithuania also shows that patients in Lithuania are less likely to forego or postpone care (17.5%) than in the EU overall (26.5%) and in neighbouring countries (38.8% in Estonia and 41.8% in Latvia).

Figure 2.11. Relatively few people declare unmet need for medical examinations and the spread between the rich and the poor is limited

Self-declared unmet need for medical examination for financial, geographic or waiting times reasons, by income quintile, 2015

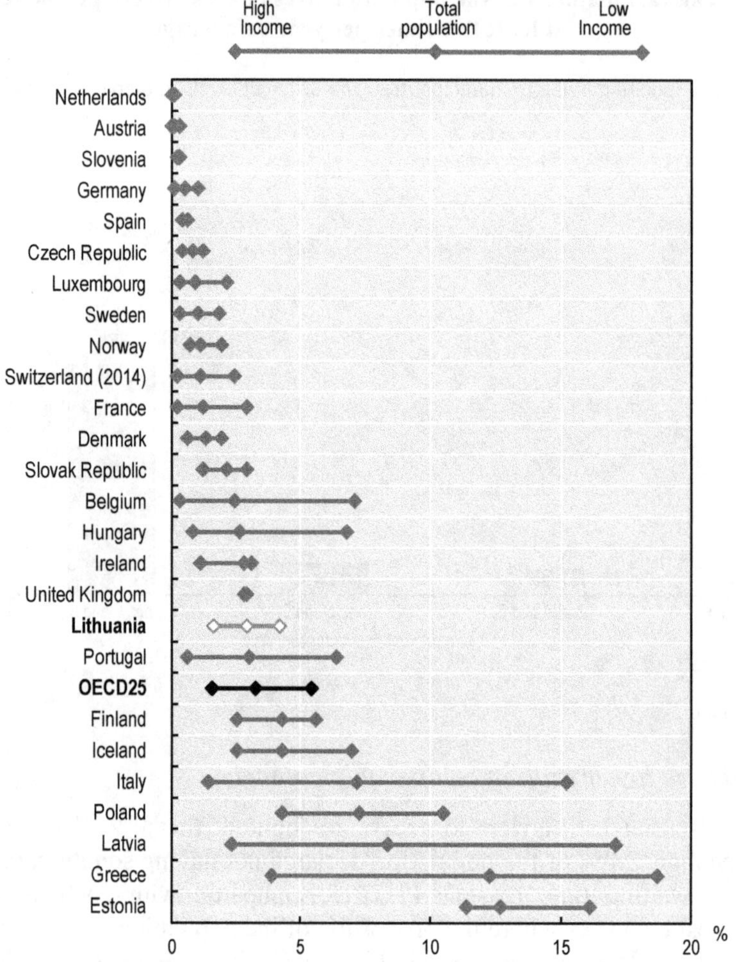

Source: Eurostat Database, based on EU-SILC.

Few Lithuanians in particular perceive financial barriers to access. In Lithuania, only 2% of the population declared having foregone medical care for financial reasons in the 2014 EHIS (Table 2.1). The proportion foregoing dental care (which is generally considered to be more price-elastic) was 5%, but only 2% for prescribed pharmaceuticals, which is perhaps surprising given the extensive out-of-pocket payments on medicines. People in the second income quintile clearly feel the pressure on their finances more than the rest of the population, including those in the first quintile, but overall inequalities are not very pronounced. The SILC survey also point to the fact that cost is not the main reason for unmet needs.

Table 2.1. Proportion of the population for which needs were not met in the past 12 months due to financial reasons, by income quintile

	Total	I	II	III	IV	V
Medical care	2	3	4	2	1	1
Dental care	5	6	10	6	3	1
Prescribed medicines	2	2	6	2	1	1

Source: Statistics Lithuania (2015) Results of the Health Interview Survey of the Population of Lithuania 2014

Relatively speaking, waiting times are much more of a constraint to access. No administrative data on waiting times are available that would enable a comparison between Lithuania and other countries. However, three-quarters of the people in Lithuania who declare having foregone medical care do so because of waiting times (SILC 2015). This represents 2% of the population, significantly above the 1% EU28 average but nevertheless below the UK (2.5%), Finland (4.2%) and Estonia (above 11%). The NHIF and territorial insurance funds monitor and publish information about waiting times for a large range of services, by municipality, type of provider, and type of surgery. Patients can search the databases and look up services provided and timeframes in different facilities and can enquire about the waiting time in a given facility[6]. They can also register on waiting lists outside their regions. Additionally, for hip and knee replacement, patients awaiting surgery are given a unique number and can trace their own progress on the list. If they want to obtain the service more quickly, they can purchase their prosthesis and progress to surgery but will only be reimbursed at the time they would have received the service for free. Pensioners can also obtain a dental prosthesis and seek reimbursement later for a pre-defined amount. In 2019 a new waiting time guarantee will come into effect.

Increasing attention will need to be paid to measuring and, as needed, addressing possible barriers in access to care. While high-level analyses suggest access to care in Lithuania is reasonable, a more nuanced understanding of the situation is required. Indeed, available data are not sufficiently detailed to assess the nature and the distribution of the financial burden people face in accessing care and particularly in obtaining medicines. Little is known about the constraints faced by those living in rural areas. While summary data on waiting times are not readily available it is likely that access to care is problematic for some groups of the population and may contribute to inequalities in outcomes. Monitoring systems need to be strengthened and measures designed to address identified issues.

2.3. For pharmaceuticals, Lithuania, like many countries, struggles to balance access and sustainability

The public coverage of retail pharmaceuticals spending remains very low in Lithuania compared with OECD countries, and the government has stepped up efforts to increase the take-up of generics (3.1) and increase the transparency of its pharmaceutical policy (3.2).

2.3.1. A more effective promotion of generics would help curb out-of-pocket payments on retail drugs

Medicines used in ambulatory care are extensively funded out-of-pocket. In Lithuania, in 2015, 68% of spending on retail pharmaceuticals, which includes over-the-counter products, was paid by patients out of pocket. This is much higher than the OECD average (37%) and higher than in all OECD countries with the exception of Latvia (also 68%). The level of out-of-pocket payments for prescribed medicines in part depends on patients' choices. The coverage rules described above foresee a payment per package (with some exceptions – see Section 2.2.1) as well as a co-payment (50, 20, 10 or 0%) based on the reference price. In addition, patients must pay the difference if the retail price of a drug is higher than the reference price, which is the case for majority of drugs in Lithuania. Since 2010 pharmacies have been required to offer at least one generic product in a group of medicines at a retail price not exceeding the reference price. Patients in fact often select non-generic drugs instead of cheaper generic alternatives, implying that some out-of-pocket payments could potentially be avoided. At the same time, the system is very complex and patients' choices may not always be fully informed.

Several measures have been implemented to improve the uptake of generics among patient population but more needs to be done to address prescriber and pharmacy practices. Since 2010, pharmacies are obliged to inform patients about the prices of medicines and to stock the cheapest generic within a group of medicines. In 2016, NHIF also conducted a public multimedia information campaign on the benefits of generics, but to date no data are available on its impact. A degree of opposition to generics appears to be common among clinicians. Since 2011, they are required to prescribe outpatient medicines by INN (International Non-proprietary Name), with some exceptions (biological medicines and composite medicines with 3 or more substances). In inpatient setting, the Medical Advisory Committee of the health care institution in question must provide an argument justifying the use of a non-generic drug.

In 2017, the government made a commitment to step up the measures supporting the adoption of generics and the rational use of medicines. The 2017 guidelines for pharmaceutical market policy stress, among others, the need to improve monitoring of prescriptions and develop e-tools to support clinicians in optimal prescribing through the already existing e-health Services and Cooperation Infrastructure Information System (ESPBI IS). Moreover, a commitment has been made to strengthen dissemination of information to the public on the rational use of medicines and to develop a 'Wise list of medicines' for clinicians (following the Swedish 'Wise List' example and the international 'Choosing Wisely' initiative) (Ministry of Health, Lithuania, 2017). At present, work on an implementation plan for these measures is being carried out.

Additional financial incentives could be introduced drawing on the experience of OECD countries. A range of pay-for-performance programmes for clinicians, linking financial incentives to prescription targets for generics, exist in the OECD countries (OECD,

2017b). Furthermore, financial incentives for pharmacies to dispense cheaper products are widely used. In Lithuania, the current regulations stipulate regressive pharmacy margins, but the rate of decrease in the margins is too low to create adequate incentive.

2.3.2. Pricing methods and reimbursement decisions help curb public costs but more transparency is required.

As many OECD countries, Lithuania relies on a range of pricing mechanisms to contain costs. As discussed in Section 2.1., the reimbursement prices (reference price) of patent-protected medicines (as well as branded off-patent medicines) are set to 95% of the average over the lowest prices in each of the eight reference countries (external reference pricing). Since 2018, the reference prices are calculated on quarterly basis. When the first generic enters the market, its price is set to 50% of the originator's price, and the second and third generic at 15% below the price of the first one[7]. In general, medicines are grouped by active ingredient (INN). Some therapies, i.e. insulins and asthma medications, are subject to higher-level clustering by indication, which allows for grouping drugs with different active ingredients (INN). The reimbursement price is based on the cheapest product available in the market within each cluster of medicines (internal reference pricing). Managed entry agreements are applied for all new patent protected products in the market. These pricing mechanisms are frequently used in OECD countries and all have advantages and drawbacks. Unsurprisingly, opinions differ about the overall adequacy of the pricing system among stakeholders (MoH and NHIF on the one hand, professional associations of industries on the other). A 2011 study comparing prices at 6-9 years after the introduction of 5 generics showed reimbursed expenditure per dose had dropped between 56 and 87% (Garuoliene et al., 2011).

In 2017, the government intensified efforts to cap retail prices and reduce user charges on outpatient medicines. As discussed in Section 2.1, the retail prices of most medicines – the prices at which medicines are offered in pharmacies – have been significantly higher than their reference prices (the prices, to which the reimbursement rates apply) with patients required to cover the difference out of pocket. This has contributed markedly to high user charges. Since July 2017, regulations stipulate that the retail price of a drug cannot exceed its reference price by more than 10%. This rule applies to clusters of medicines with a least three manufacturers. If the condition is not met, the drug cannot be included in the list of reimbursed medicines (Ministry of Health, Lithuania 2017).

The government also recognises the need to improve procurement processes for inpatient medicines. The NHIF negotiates prices and procures expensive specialty inpatient medicines many of which are introduced under managed entry agreements; these generally work well and disputes with manufacturers are rare. The procurement of basic inpatient drugs occurs either at the level of the Central Procurement Institution or by individual hospitals. In the latter case, the hospitals need to prove that the prices obtained are lower than prices negotiated by the Central Procurement. Indeed, large hospitals are frequently able to negotiate lower prices, a fact that calls into question the effectiveness of the Central Procurement. As the market in Lithuania is relatively small compared to other EU Member States, the government recognizes that measures at national level are not sufficient to ensure accessibility of medicines and sustainability of the pharmaceutical care budget. As a result the 2017 guidelines for pharmaceutical market policy also include a commitment to establishing international cooperation in procurement, in particular in medicines for rare diseases (Ministry of Health, Lithuania, 2017). To further support long-term sustainability, it will also be important to recognise the need for the procurement strategies to differ across segments of the market depending on the patent status of a drug and number of substitutable patent-protected or off-patent medicines (OECD, 2017b).

Steps have been taken recently to improve the transparency of reimbursement decisions and earmark specific funds for new drugs. Decisions to include new drugs on the reimbursement list are made by the MoH, factoring in the recommendations of the Reimbursement Committee, the Compulsory Health Insurance Council and the NHIF. Since 2011, in an effort to improve access to novel drugs, the savings obtained from the pricing measures described above have been reinvested to finance access to new medicines. Most stakeholders agree that the decision process about the inclusion of new drugs lacks transparency and that prioritisation is perhaps more politically driven than evidence-based. Important steps to address this were taken in 2016, in particular: reimbursement decisions must be made within 180 days; new qualifications and experience requirements for the members of Reimbursement Committee have been imposed and decision criteria publicly reported. Moreover, the 2017 guidelines for pharmaceutical market policy envisage shortening 'waiting times' for moving new medicines from the so-called 'reserve list' to the list of reimbursed medicines, from 1 year (in 2016) to 6 months (in 2020), and to 3 months (in 2027) (Ministry of Health, Lithuania, 2017). Whether this can be achieved and the budget impact of these measures remain open questions.

Health technology assessment (HTA) capacity still needs to be strengthened. While reimbursement and pricing decision processes are structured, they remain insufficiently based on HTA. Lithuania has sought to address this problem, rather unsuccessfully, since 1993 (Wild et al., 2015). More recently (between 2013 and 2015), two organisations under the Ministry of Health were working on HTA capacity building but the results remain unclear. Efforts must be sustained to build a solid foundation for rational and transparent decisions. At the same time, given Lithuania's size, every opportunity should be seized to take part in international collaborations in these matters. The above-mentioned guidelines for pharmaceutical market policy include further commitment to strengthening HTA capacity in the country by adapting best international practices and through international cooperation (for example, within EUnetHTA) (Ministry of Health, Lithuania, 2017).

Lithuania needs a more explicit national medicines policy. Lithuania is a rather small market in which regulations change frequently. This can undermine the industry's business confidence and the authorities' ability to negotiate with them and ensure sustainable availability of medicines. The development and promulgation of a comprehensive national medicines policy could help in that respect. The policy should lay out clear objectives and priorities addressing financing, individual and collective affordability, technical and allocative efficiency, and long-term sustainability. Stakeholders should contribute to its development and commit to supporting it once agreed. The guidelines for pharmaceutical market policy, adopted by the government in 2017, are a promising step in the direction of more effective policies.

Conclusion

On balance, the overall assessment of the performance of Lithuania's health system on the key dimensions of sustainability and access is rather positive. Lithuania's spending on health is low and efforts to keep public spending in check are effective. At the same time, the sustainability of the system is not only a matter of public finance. Improving health outcomes and the financial protection of the population is likely to require additional investments. Nevertheless, people have reasonable access to the system and unmet needs are lower than in countries with comparable income and spending. This balance – as everywhere – is a difficult one to maintain. In particular, more needs to be done to protect people from high out-of-pocket spending on pharmaceuticals and to ensure that additional funds invested in the system are geared towards improving the lagging outcomes described in chapter 1. As chapter 3 will show, efforts in particular will need to be stepped up to increase the efficiency and quality of services delivered.

Notes

1. Contributions for farmers, self-employed, self-insured, beneficiaries of specific pensions etc. are computed differently.

2. In fact, official population statistics for 2016 give a total population of 2.88 million and the number of insured registered is 2.93 million – which highlights difficulties in determining the true size of the population and thus the number of uninsured.

3. In 2015, the Agency in charge of collecting social contributions recovered contributions from around 94,000 insured people in Lithuania, three quarters of which were self-employed and around 13% farmers.

4. In Lithuania, as a general rule medicines are grouped according to International Non-proprietary Name (INN), which indicates the type of the active ingredient in the drug. A few exceptions from this rule are discussed in Section 2.3.

5. The eight reference countries are countries with GDP per capita comparable with Lithuania, i.e. Bulgaria, Czech Republic, Estonia, Hungary, Latvia, Poland, Slovakia, and Romania.

6. In March 2017, 41 facilities were listed as providing hip-knee replacement in Lithuania. The waiting time ranged from 0 to 25 months at Vilnius University hospital. It was a year or more in 5 facilities, 3 of which in Vilnius and the other in each of the 2 main cities.

7. If there are four or more products with the same active substance as identified by INN (International Non-proprietary Name), the price of the most expensive product cannot exceed the price of the cheapest one by more than 40 % (reduced from 50% in 2011), Information provided by the Ministry of Health, Lithuania (2016).

References

European Commission (2015), The 2015 Ageing Report: Economic and Budgetary Projections for the 28 EU Countries (2015-2060), *European Economy Series*, No. 3.

European Commission (2017), Corruption, *Special Eurobarometer 470*, October.

Garuoliene K., et al. (2011, "European countries with small populations can obtain low prices for drugs: Lithuania as a case history.' *Expert review of pharmacoeconomics & outcomes research*, Vol 11, pp. 343–349.

Habibov, N, and A. Cheung (2017), "Revisiting informal payments in 29 transitional countries: The scale and socio-economic correlates", *Social Science & Medicine*, Vol. 178, Issue C, pp. 28-37.

Kacevičius, G. and M. Karanikolos (2015). "The impact of the financial crisis on the health system and health in Lithuania" in Maresso, A. et al., eds. *Economic crisis, health systems and health in Europe: country experience*, WHO Regional Office for Europe/European Observatory on Health Systems and Policies, Copenhagen.

Ministry of Health, Lithuania (2017), Medicines Policy Guidelines (unofficial translation into English).

Murauskienė, L. and S. Thomson (2018), Can people afford to pay for health care? New evidence on financial protection in Lithuania, WHO Regional Office for Europe, Copenhagen.

NICE – National Institute for Health and Care Excellence (2014) Clinical guideline [CG181] Cardiovascular disease: risk assessment and reduction, including lipid modification, Clinical guideline [CG181], Last updated: September 2016, https://www.nice.org.uk/guidance/cg181.

OECD/European Observatory on Health Systems and Policies (2017), *Lithuania: Country Health Profile 2017*, OECD Publishing, Paris/European Observatory on Health Systems and Policies, Brussels, http://dx.doi.org/10.1787/9789264283473-en.

OECD (2017), *Health at a Glance 2017: OECD Indicators*, OECD Publishing, Paris, http://dx.doi.org/10.1787/health_glance-2017-en.

OECD (2017b), *Tackling Wasteful Spending on Health*, OECD Publishing, Paris, http://dx.doi.org/10.1787/9789264266414-en

Statistics Lithuania (2015) Results of the Health Interview Survey of the Population of Lithuania 2014 Lietuvos statistikos departamentas, Vilnius. https://osp.stat.gov.lt/services-portlet/pub-edition-file?id=20908.

Wild C, et al (2015) Background Analysis for National HTA Strategy for Lithuania. Focus on Medical Devices. Decision Support Document No. 90 ; 2015. Vienna: Ludwig Boltzmann Institute for Health Technology Assessment.

Chapter 3. Health care system in Lithuania: Efficiency and quality

This chapter assesses the efficiency and quality of health care in Lithuania. Given its income and investment in health, comparisons consistently show that Lithuania could be achieving better health outcomes. The necessary adaptation of service delivery is well under way. Primary health care is given a large responsibility in managing the population's health and its organisation emulates best OECD practices. Progress towards the rationalisation of the hospital sector has been slower and recent efforts to improve public health and to control risk factors must be sustained. In recent years, an increasing number of measures have sought to improve quality. Overall, results have improved, sometimes rapidly, but Lithuania often remains on par with low-performing OECD countries.

The statistical data for Israel are supplied by and under the responsibility of the relevant Israeli authorities. The use of such data by the OECD is without prejudice to the status of the Golan Heights, East Jerusalem and Israeli settlements in the West Bank under the terms of international law.

Introduction

High-level analyses suggest significant scope for improving the efficiency and quality, in particular the effectiveness, of service delivery in Lithuania. Even though life expectancy is rising in Lithuania, it does not meet the levels which can be expected relative to income (GDP) and health spending levels. Several other central European and OECD countries with the same level of health spending and income have a considerably higher life expectancy (Figure 3.1). These findings were confirmed by a European Commission study analysing the relative efficiency of European countries which related both life expectancy and amenable mortality to various indicators of system resources, financial as well as human and physical. The results consistently show that Lithuania has one of the highest potential gains in health outcomes given the resources used (Medeiros and Schwierz, 2015). In Lithuania, both preventable and amenable mortality are high compared to other European countries. This means the Lithuanian life expectancy should improve both by reducing risk factors like smoking, alcohol and traffic, and by improved effectiveness in the services provided.

Figure 3.1. Many countries with comparable level of income and health spending as Lithuania achieve better outcomes

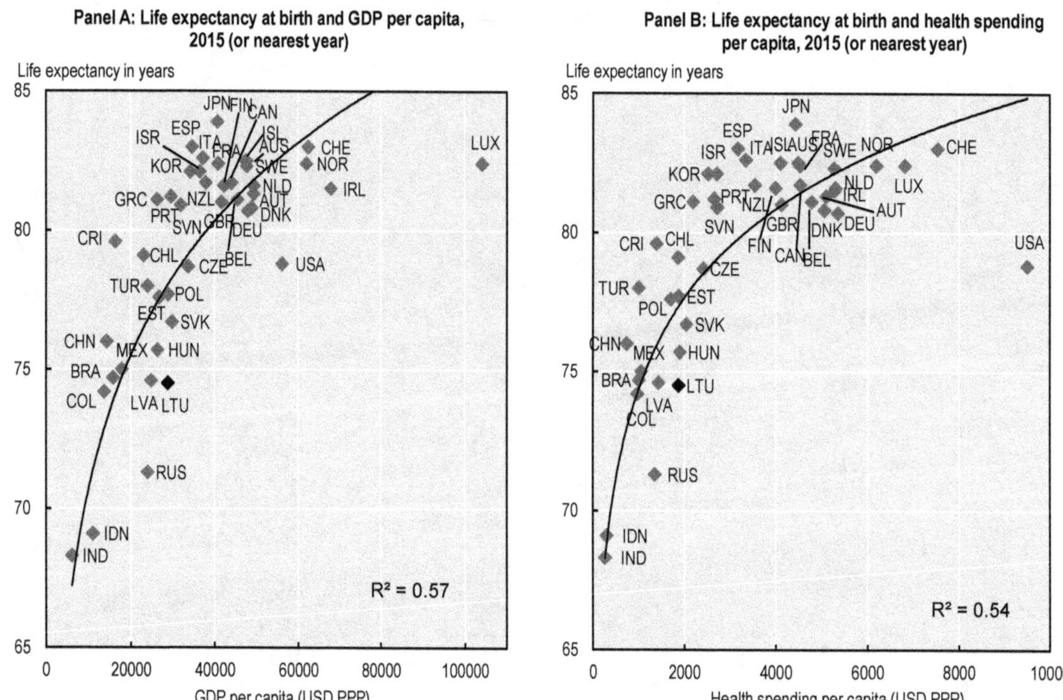

Source: OECD Health Statistics 2017, http://dx.doi.org/10.1787/health-data-en (data refers to 2015).

In order to refine this initial diagnostic and suggest ways forward, this third chapter analyses the policies in place to increase efficiency (3.1) and quality (3.2) and assesses the current performance of Lithuania in this regard.

3.1. Efforts in rebalancing service delivery must be pursued and deepened to increase efficiency.

The question under consideration here is whether the Lithuanian health system is organised in a way which is conducive to maximising value for money. Rebalancing service delivery and investing in public health are key elements of Lithuania's strategy in this regard. Prior to 1990, the role of primary health care and health promotion was limited and services were predominantly delivered in a range of hospitals, which were numerous and frequently narrowly specialised by disease or population segment. Reorganising the hospital sector and reducing its size, rebalancing service delivery in favour of a modernised and considerably strengthened primary care and developing better strategies to tackle risk factors have been the main drivers behind service delivery reforms in Eastern and central Europe since transition. Lithuania is no exception and all stakeholders have been consistently aligned behind these priorities.

This section describes how Lithuania has reshaped its health service delivery system to adapt the role of hospitals and fundamentally modernised primary health care (PHC), and points to areas which need further development. It also reviews mental health and efforts to strengthen public health.

3.1.1. Lithuania's steady efforts to overhaul the hospital sector need to be pursued

Lithuania has achieved a substantial reconfiguration of its hospital system

The current configuration of the hospital system represents progress in shaping the hospital sector. In 2015, there were 119 public hospitals (legal entities), which represents a considerable drop from the 1991 level of 202. The number of monoprofile hospitals has substantially decreased (from 39 in 2001 to 14 in 2015), through closures or administrative integration with general hospitals (there is only one self-standing TB facility and no administratively independent infectious diseases hospitals). The MoH manages 10 "republican level" facilities which are generally large (700 beds) and there are 49 smaller municipal hospitals (180 beds on average). The private sector includes 10 small inpatient facilities, a handful of specialised facilities and seven outpatient surgery centres (Table 3.1).

Many countries have been more effective in consolidating hospital infrastructure. Despite the progress noted, Lithuania still has a very large number of hospitals, with at least one in almost every municipality and a high number of beds. Since 1992, more than half of the beds have been closed through administratively planned downsizing and application of incentives such as shifting the funding to an output based reimbursement. However, most of this reduction took place in the 1990s. The number of beds has continuously declined. Nevertheless, Lithuania's fast shrinking population led to increases in number of beds per capita during the years 2000s, so today Lithuania remains with Germany, Austria and Hungary among the European countries with the most hospital beds. Compared to neighbouring Baltic countries, the pace of change in reducing hospital capacity has been relatively slow: between 2000 and 2015, the number of beds in Latvia dropped by 54%, in Estonia by 42% and in Lithuania 27% (Figure 3.2).

Table 3.1. Number of hospitals in Lithuania, 2015

Hospitals	Number of legal entities		Number of functional entities*		Average size and activity	
	Public	Private	Public	Private	Beds	Discharges/year
General, of which	61	5	65	5	265	9928
Republican-level subordinated to MoH	10		13		717	30037
Republican-level subordinated to other Ministries	2		2		130	2878
Municipal	49		50		177	5816
Private		5		5	25	1582
Specialised, of which	14	2	23	2	153	2563
Psychiatric	4	2	6	2	208	2221
Substance abuse	5		5		47	891
Tuberculosis	1		5		119	395
Oncology	1		2		271	10438
Infectious diseases			1		52	2657
Maternity	1		1		152	7396
Rehab	2		3		192	2982
Nursing	44	3	48	3	59	327
Total	119	10	136	10	174	5313
Outpatient surgery centres		7		7		

Note: a number specialised facilities were formerly self-standing but are now administratively integrated within general hospitals, hence a higher number of functional than legal entities.
Source: Ministry of Health, Lithuania.

Figure 3.2. The number of hospital beds has slowly declined and remains high

Hospital beds per 1 000 population, 2000 and 2015

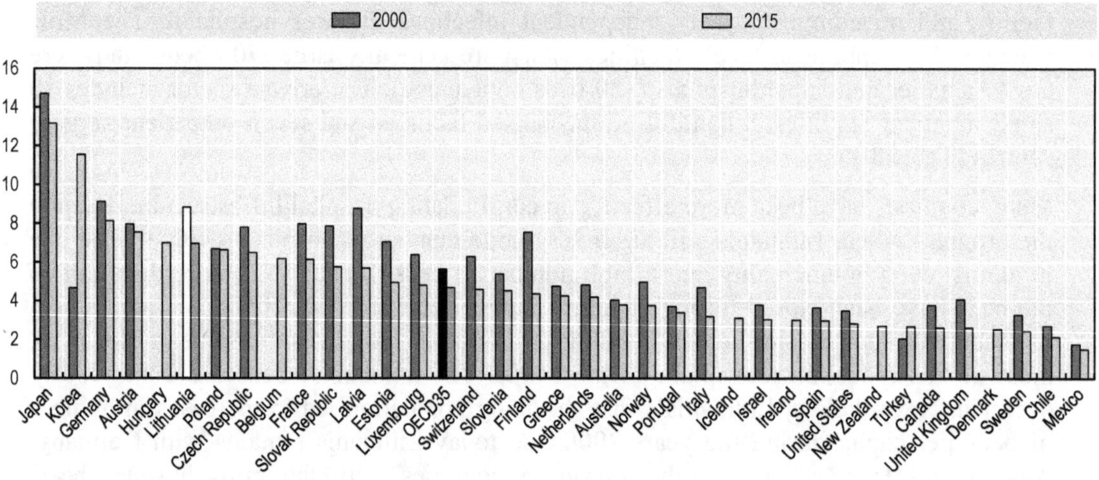

Source: OECD Health Statistics 2017, http://dx.doi.org/10.1787/health-data-en.

There is still room to further rationalise the hospital sector

Average lengths of stay average are relatively short with a notable exception. The average length of stay (ALOS) for curative care, at 6.3 days (2015), compares well internationally and is below the OECD average (6.7). But this number has not progressed the last five years. Tuberculosis stands out as one diagnostic area in which Lithuania has distinctively long treatment lengths. Long length of stays corresponds to a traditional and some would argue outdated inpatient mode of treatment for TB which characterises many former Soviet countries. Nonetheless, at 102 days (2015), Lithuania ALOS is twice as high as most Baltic neighbours and Central European countries, and compares poorly with the OECD average of 24 days.

The low and very variable bed occupancy rate indicates the hospital sector remains in overcapacity. In 2015, among the 65 public general hospitals, the average bed occupancy rate was 73.5% (or 268 days per year), which is below the OECD average of 77%. There are however large variations among general hospitals (Figure 3.3) with predominantly small hospitals reporting very low rates. This means that many beds are not used at all. The current health system development plan aims to increased bed occupancy levels and sets a target of 300 days per year (above 82%). In 2015, only 4 of the 65 public general hospitals in Lithuania met this target. In fact, the bed occupancy rate was lower than 60% in 13 public hospitals.

Figure 3.3. The acute care bed occupancy ratio is lower than the OECD average in 85% of Lithuanian hospitals

Bed Occupancy rate of public general hospital, 2015

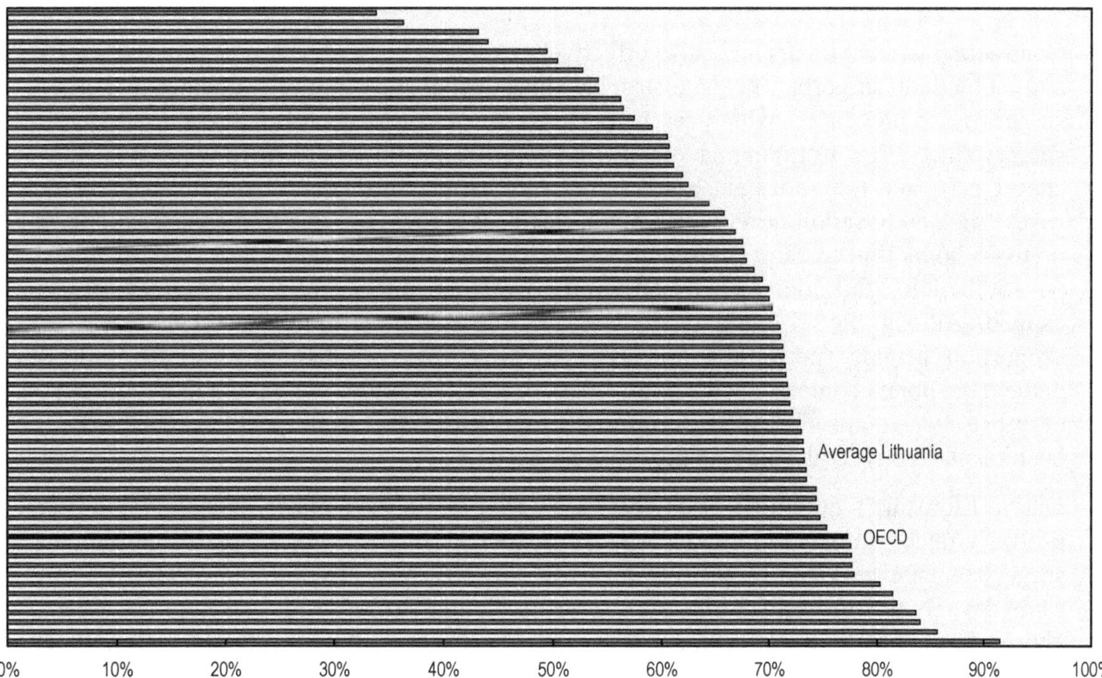

Source: Ministry of Health, Lithuania.

Payment systems and contracting methods have been increasingly leveraged to encourage more efficient modes of delivery

DRGs combined with volume caps seek to encourage efficient delivery and lower volumes of inpatient hospitalisations. In 2012, a DRG system based on the Australian coding and diagnosis grouping was introduced and continues to be fine-tuned. For example, Lithuania is developing new cost weights to ensure relative prices reflect more closely the local cost structure of service production. The DRG system allows payments to hospitals to mirror their patients' case-mix and incentivises the more efficient production of treatment episodes. It can also potentially encourage increases in the number of hospitalisations. In order to counteract this incentive, contracts between the NHIF with individual facilities include volume ceilings for in-patient services which are decreased year-on-year. Some services, such as the care of children under age three, obstetrics and specific acute procedures are not capped though. Additionally:

- To encourage reductions in volumes without penalising hospitals with proportionally reduced budgets, if the volume of a specific inpatient service is below the amount agreed in the contract, the price index for the service is increased and the hospital can receive at least part of the initially planned budget for the given year (but no more).
- If the volume of a specific inpatient service is more than 10% above the national average in a given area, no new contracts can be signed with additional providers (conversely, new contracts can be signed if the exiting volume is 10% below the national average).
- For all services, if volumes exceed the contractual volumes, additional cases are reimbursed at a lower rate.

Contracting and payments have also effectively encouraged the development of day-cases and outpatient surgery. The Ministry has introduced and regularly updates a list of surgeries and procedures which can be performed as day-cases since 2007 and outpatient surgery since 2013. In Lithuania, outpatient surgeries are those performed without general anaesthesia, and they are paid based on a price-list established by the Ministry. "Day-cases" include hospitalisation which are typically less than 24 hours but can be extended up to 48 hours if necessary. In order to encourage their development, since 2012, they are paid at the DRG full price. In addition, for individual hospitals, day-cases volumes are not capped. Among the 71 main procedures eligible to be performed as day-cases, the proportion actually performed as day-cases was 58% in 2016, an increase of 20 percentage points compared with 2012. In 2016, tonsillectomies were included in the day-case list and around 45% were performed as day cases that same year. In other words, hospitals are actively developing the day-case activity.

Due to Lithuania's definition of day-cases, its progress in developing shorter surgeries is probably underestimated in international comparisons. International standards define day surgery as care provided to patients formally admitted to a hospital and discharged the same day. By this measure, Lithuania is very much lagging behind in developing modern approaches to hospital treatment, but the picture looks very different if the local definition of "day case" is used. For instance, while 0.3% of Laparoscopic cholecystectomy were carried out on an ambulatory basis by international statistical standards, a level similar to most Central European countries, nearly 36% were conducted in day-surgery – and patients released within 48 hours (Figure 3.4).

Figure 3.4. Lithuania has probably been better at developing efficient surgeries than international statistics suggest

Share of Laparoscopic cholecystectomy carried out as day-surgery cases, 2015 (or nearest years)

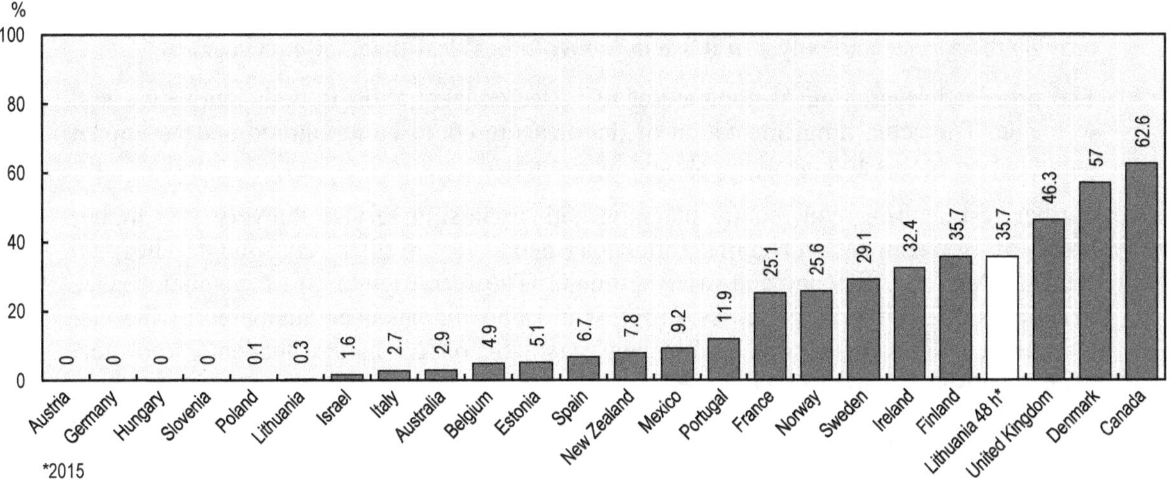

Source: NHIF and OECD Health Statistics, http://dx.doi.org/10.1787/health-data-en.

Further consolidation of service delivery is warranted on efficacy and safety grounds and steps have been taken in that direction.

Surgeries are carried out in the vast majority of hospitals in Lithuania, which is inefficient and also carries a risk for patients. Of the 65 hospitals with a general profile contracted by the NHIF, 52 provided at least one surgical procedure in the year. Among them 22 carried out less than 250 procedures, which is roughly one per (business) day. Moreover, the number and complexity of these procedures varies considerably across hospitals, and many carry out major surgeries at very low frequency, for instance:

- 45 hospitals undertook appendectomy, but 23 of these performed appendectomies less than once a week;
- 37 hospitals conducted hysterectomies or C-sections, but among them 15 undertook any one of these major obstetric intervention less than once a week;
- 24 hospitals performed hip surgery, but while 5 performed them less than once a week, the 7 busiest one did more than 11 such surgeries per week.

In the vast majority of cases, these surgeries can be programmed. Concentrating their delivery in a few places could allow a more efficient use of staff and equipment. More importantly, the fact that so many facilities carry out few surgeries raises serious concerns about their capacity to deliver good outcomes.

The decision to use minimum volume thresholds for contracting is a bold step in the right direction. Lithuania intends on concentrating services in fewer places and is using volume targets for obstetrics and common surgeries in contracting to that effect. Since 2016, the plan is that unless a hospital is more than 50km away from the nearest one, or it has recently received specific investments, it will no longer be contracted by the NHIF when if carries out fewer than 300 births per year or less than 400 major surgeries. In 2015, half of the public general hospitals in Lithuania (31 of 65) had an obstetric department. In 14 of these, less than 300 deliveries were conducted.

There is evidence that concentration can be achieved in Lithuania: transluminal coronary angioplasties are only carried out in 5 public hospitals, on a very large scale, and less than two times a week in a private facility. Cataract surgery is also concentrated: 12 hospitals provide the service and only 4 of those in low volumes (less than 150 in a year).

The proposed leveraging of contracting to foster concentration is both innovative and welcome. The actual implementation of the measure could be monitored and its impact including on access and outcomes should be evaluated.

Further restructuring will require planning and organising service delivery at a higher level of government. Overall, Lithuania needs to further consolidate hospital infrastructure on efficiency and safety grounds. The reconfiguration of hospital service delivery is difficult in all countries. Progress in Lithuania has been hampered by the fact that municipalities, which own and manage hospitals, have a natural tendency to protect local interests, in terms of perceived access to services or simply employment. Many countries in the wider Europe region have realised that the distribution of hospitals services needs to be decided at a higher level than the municipality. In Finland, hospital boards jointly manage several municipal hospitals, and the soon to be created counties will actually be responsible for jointly planning and coordinating service delivery across all health and social care previously delivered by municipalities. Austria, Denmark and Croatia have also re-concentrated the responsibility for planning and organising hospital service delivery at increasingly higher levels of government. Sweden is considering a consolidation of administrative levels. Similarly, the reorganisation of hospital service delivery will also need to be decided and governed across sets of municipalities. This might require a formal national service plan to be formulated. In addition, the governance and ownership framework of hospitals may need to be adapted to enable and incentivise reorganisation of service delivery across municipal and possibly regional boundaries.

3.1.2. Lithuania has developed a modern primary health care system

Lithuania clearly recognises that a strong primary health care is the foundation of a health system that is effective, efficient and responsive to patients' needs and has developed the system accordingly.

The number of trained general practitioners is now higher than in many OECD countries. As other former Soviet republics, Lithuania inherited a policlinics-based PHC sector in which frontline services were delivered by internists, gynaecologists and paediatricians. General practice was introduced as a clinical and licensed specialty in the nineties and the workforce has increased rapidly. In 2015, GPs represented 83% of primary care physician workforce in Lithuania (versus 7% in 1998 and 60% in 2000). Today, the number of GPs per population is higher in Lithuania than in most OECD countries (Figure 3.5). Where GPs are not available, teams of specialists (internist, paediatrician, gynaecologist, and surgeon) continue to jointly deliver primary care.

Figure 3.5. Lithuania has consistently increased the number of GPs in the health system

Number of GPs per 1 000 population, OECD countries and Lithuania

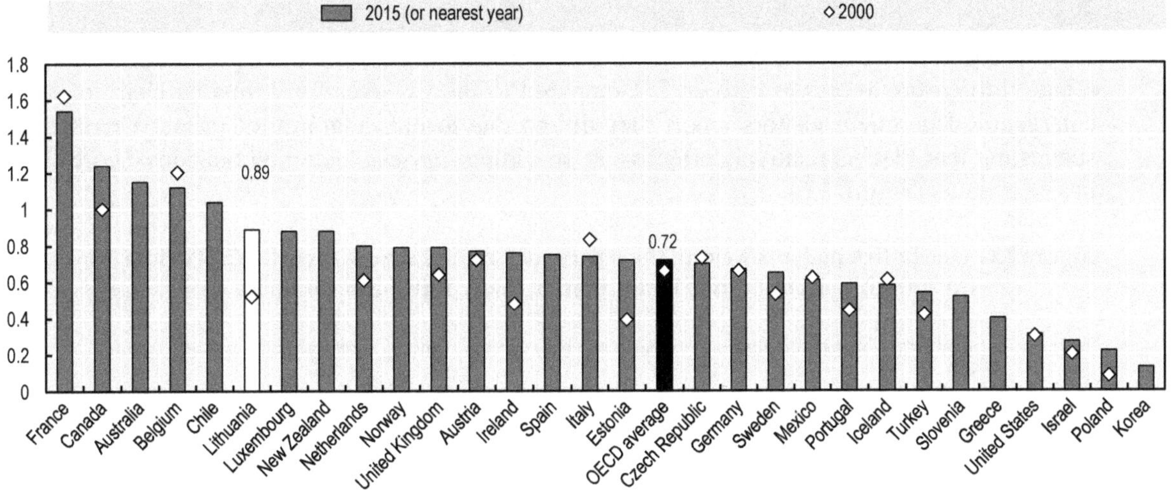

Source: OECD Health Statistics 2017, http://dx.doi.org/10.1787/health-data-en.

Nurses are an inherent part of the PHC workforce and their role is continuously expanding. A primary care team contracted by the NHIF must include a primary care or community nurse. Since 2015, nurses can prescribe medical aids (under physician supervision) and have been given a greater role in providing services to chronic patients with non-communicable diseases (lifestyle counselling, self-care and monitoring of health status during checks-ups). A few (75) primary health care facilities also employ diabetes nurses who provide diabetic foot care, lifestyle counselling, self-care and monitoring of health status[1]. Nurses can undertake home visits (paid on top of the capitation) and since 2016 can be independently contracted by the territorial insurance funds to that effect. In 2015, a two-year master's degree for advanced practice nursing was introduced and the new graduates are also expected to take an increasing role in primary care for of chronic patients, as well as anaesthesiology-intensive care and emergency care.

Primary care services are delivered in a variety of public and private settings remunerated through a mixed but predominantly capitation-based system. Most PHC facilities are owned by the municipalities but private clinics can open and work on the same terms as public. In cities, polyclinics also include outpatient specialists. In remote areas public facilities can also run community medical dispensaries to bring services closer to the population. Public facilities are typically larger entities: they represent 39% of PHC providers but cover around 70% of the population. Public and private providers are all contracted and monitored the same way. A little less than ¾ of their remuneration comes from a capitation adjusted for age and they receive additional payments to incentivise quality (see next section). In effect, the majority of PHC is provided by publically employed GPs working in groups, while some clinics in terms of staffing look like traditional polyclinics.

Primary care providers have been given a key role in managing patients' health. Virtually the entire population is registered with a GP or a primary care team. Gatekeeping was introduced in 2002. Patients cannot obtain free PHC services unless they are registered with a GP and referrals are required for specialised care in most cases. PHC providers are financially incentivised to deliver specific services and expected to coordinate patient care. They must also be informed about care provided by others (specialists, hospitals). The number of PHC visits per person per year has increased from 4.8 in 2007 to 5.7 in 2014.

PHC providers effectively contribute to the continuity of care. PHC providers are required to ensure access to care 24/7. Compared to the EU average, a smaller share of emergency department visitors report they did so due to unavailability of primary care, suggesting that PHC is relatively effective at providing services including outside of core business hours (Figure 3.6).

Figure 3.6. One in five patients went to the emergency room because their PHC provider was unavailable, but this is better than in many European countries

Share of patients who visited an emergency department because the primary care physician was not available

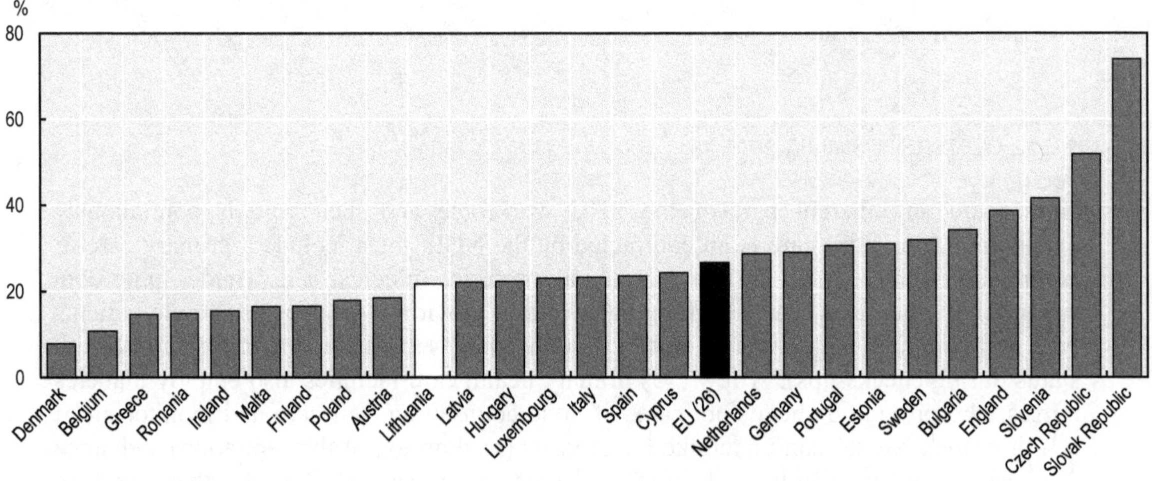

Source: van den Berg et al. (2016)

GPs' role could be further strengthened in some areas, on efficiency but also quality grounds. The delineation of responsibilities between GPs and specialist needs to further evolve. GPs believe that some guidelines continue to unnecessarily limit their responsibilities. For some chronic diseases (e.g. diabetes, cardiovascular diseases), the PHC doctor is obliged to refer the patient to a specialist once per year. After the first visit, patients can choose to go to the specialist directly for further monitoring and treatment. In other cases (type 2 diabetes for children, asthma) guidelines further specify conditions for referral or limit GPs' scope of practice. In the absence of evidence of the effectiveness of these strategies, a case can be made that such mandatory referrals effectively take the responsibility for case management away from the GP and signal that the PHC cannot take responsibility.

3.1.3. Lithuania needs to further strengthen mental health services and curb suicide incidence

Awareness is high about mental health problems, as shown by the many strategies developed to respond to the problem. The 1998-2010 National Health Programme had several specific mental health objectives, some of which were implemented, such as the development of municipal Mental Health Centres. In 2007, the Lithuanian Mental Health Strategy outlined several guiding policies to create effective local services in primary care, schools and social services, including strengthening the role of general practitioners (GPs) in the provision of mental healthcare. The *State programme for development of public health care in municipalities 2007-2010* led to the creation of the Public Health Bureaus network, which is also responsible for the promotion of mental health and prevention of mental disorders. More recently, the strengthening of mental health services was one of five objectives laid out in the health programme of the government adopted by Parliament in December 2016 (Parliament of the Republic of Lithuania, 2016).

In line with its strategies, Lithuania has reformed the service delivery structure for mental health services. Over the last 15 years, Lithuania has moved a substantial part of the institutionalised psychiatric and substance abuse services into general hospitals and outpatient mental health centres. At the same time, with investments, infrastructure conditions have improved in many psychiatric wards and departments. At the primary care level, services are delivered in 115 mental healthcare centers (MHC), which are sometimes co-located with PHC centers. MHCs are funded though capitation by the NHIF. Patients can be referred to primary level mental health services by their GP or the hospital, but also access directly.

Services in MHCs are delivered by multi-disciplinary teams of mental health workers but the workforce needs to be further developed. MHCs are meant to include psychiatrists, mental health nurses, psychologists and social workers. However, the recruitment of personnel, notably psychologists and particularly in rural areas is difficult. In 2016, there were 90 psychologists for 115 centres and geographic imbalances are a chronic problem (European Commission, 2013). In practice, the availability of services is limited: a study by the National Audit Office (2017) found, for instance, that 31% of the surveyed mental health centres staff worked less than five hours per day. Additionally, the regulations (including licensing) and guidelines surrounding psychology and psychotherapy are incomplete, the use of structured diagnostic tools limited and cognitive behavioral therapy seldom available.

Poor coordination among institutions is recognised as a major issue. The availability and proximity of mental health and primary care services does not systematically translate into a functional team approach and effective mechanisms to detect illness and meet the patients' needs. The majority of GPs state they would like to collaborate more with mental health specialists (Jaruseviciene et al, 2014). Coordination between hospital and outpatient care is also insufficient which might contribute to explaining why the suicide rate one year after hospitalisation among patients diagnosed with a mental disorder (0.73 per 100 patients) is substantially among the highest reported in the OECD.

In 2017, the National Audit Office called for renewed efforts to identify and support individuals at risk and ensure immediate and continuous support to people who have attempted suicide and emphasised the need for information sharing between institutions about individuals at risk (National Audit Office, 2017).

Primary care staff need more training and tools to fulfil their task and manage the large responsibility they have been given. Primary care should be able to play a large role in provision of mental health for patients with mild and moderate disorders. But several Lithuanian studies show that mental health issues are poorly identified and managed in primary care (Bunevicius et al., 2014 and Peceliuniene J., 2011). In contrast to the strategy to meet a larger share of mental health problems on the primary care level, GPs feel inadequately prepared to address the problem. Even if GPs feel the responsibility to manage patients' mental conditions, a direct referral to a psychiatrist or psychologist is the most common action. GPs have low confidence in the field of mental health. Only 8.8% of GPs agree with the statement "My knowledge in mental healthcare is sufficient", although rural as well as younger GPs express larger confidence in engaging in the mental healthcare of their patients (Jaruseviciene et al., 2014). Additional efforts are required to increase the capacity of the primary care system to recognise, treat and manage common mental disorders and increase access to psychological treatments.

More broadly, Lithuania could consider undertaking a systematic assessment of the current mental health service delivery system, focusing in particular on the effectiveness of - and coordination between - mental health care teams, inpatient psychiatric facilities and other segments of the health care system, including primary care. This should help identify a way forward.

3.1.4. Public health policies must be strengthened

Measures to reduce harmful alcohol consumption have been considerably strengthened recently and their effectiveness will need to be monitored

The main challenges with regard to the state of public health are well recognised. The populations' health status and behaviours indicate a sizeable room for improvement. The 2014-2025 Lithuanian Health Strategy specifies concrete goals with regard to reducing harmful alcohol consumption, tobacco, drugs and psychoactive substances, as well as encouraging healthy nutrition and physical activity. The Strategy has an impressive cross-sectorial framework (involving nearly all Ministries), and the MoH is responsible for monitoring of the implementation. The intermediate evaluation of the progress is due in 2020.

Lithuania has intensified measures to tackle the exceptionally high alcohol consumption. At the national level, the alcohol control law was amended in 2014, and new restrictions were introduced in 2016, for instance, banning the sale of alcohol products in gas stations. The tightening of alcohol legislation was one of the priorities of the government elected in 2016. In June 2017, the parliament approved the introduction of multiple alcohol restrictions, which came into effect 1st of January 2018. From this date Lithuania has a full ban on alcohol advertisement on TV, radio and internet. Alcohol sales hours were shortened by two hours in the morning and two in the evening and are now only allowed from 10 a.m. to 8 p.m. Monday to Saturday, with further restrictions Sundays. The minimum legal age for buying and consuming alcoholic beverages has been extended from 18 to 20 years. In the new legislation, retailers are responsible for controlling the age of buyers, and local governments given increased authority to limit and control sales hours in both shops and restaurants. Caterers, bars and restaurants are not limited by the time restrictions, but from 2020 further restrictions on sales come into effect, including limitations of out-door sales, for example a ban of sales on beaches, and a 7.5% alcohol limit on beverages sold during public events.

Tax increases were modest until 2017 and alcohol has become more affordable over time. Alcohol taxes (excise rates per hectolitre of pure alcohol) have been raised several times since 2000 but the increases have been low and sporadic. Between 2001 and 2008 the excise rate was even kept constant in nominal terms on beer and high alcohol-content beverages and from 2008 until 2016 increases were marginal. The prices of alcoholic beverages in Lithuania are 9% below the EU average (2016) and while food prices in Lithuania have tended to converge with average EU prices, the prices of alcohol have been more slow to do so and in fact diverged from the EU average between 2008 and 2015 (Eurostat, 2017). To put another perspective on this question of affordability, Lithuanians have experienced large increases in real wages over the last two decades, with the exception of a few years around the financial crises, while the prices of alcohol have increased much more slowly (Figure 3.7). As a consequence, alcohol affordability in Lithuania has increased substantially. Between 1996 and 2004 Lithuania had the largest increase in alcohol affordability among today's EU countries, mostly driven by a real wage increase (Rabinovich, L. et al., 2009). However, in parallel with other restrictive policies on alcohol, Lithuania raised most alcohol excise rates in March 2017 substantially, e.g. from 336 to 711 Euros per hectolitre pure alcohol on beer (MoH).

Figure 3.7. Wage in Lithuania have increased much faster than the prices of alcoholic beverages

Price indices for food, alcohol beverages and wage rates 2000-2017 (2000=100).

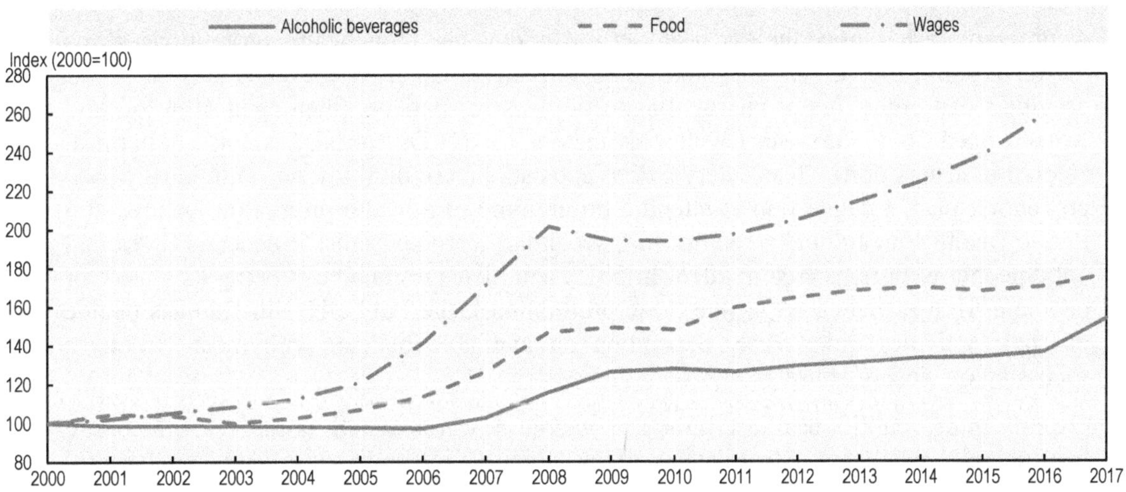

Source: Wage rates; International Financial Statistics, IMF. Food and alcohol; Eurostat (Harmonised Index of Consumer Prices).

Pricing policies and advertising regulations can be effective and cost-saving strategies to reduce harmful use of alcohol. However, restrictions in alcohol advertising are increasingly challenged by the spread of advertising on Internet, including social media (Sassi, 2015). More broadly, the degree to which alcohol use-related policies are enforced in practice is of utmost importance. After the recent changes in legislation and increase in excise rates, Lithuania should carefully monitor and evaluate enforcement level of these policies already in place before designing and implementing any new solutions. If enforcement is weak, restrictions on access and raised legal purchase age from 18 to 20 years can be inefficient at best, or at worst, lead to further development of the black market, already very high in Lithuania.

Additional gains in health and life expectancy can be obtained through interventions targeting heavy drinkers. Brief interventions typically targeting high-risk drinkers in primary care settings have been found the most effective in other OECD countries (Sassi, 2015). Although they are expensive to implement, they become cost-effective several years after their implementation. Similarly, drug and psychosocial therapy of alcohol dependence and worksite-based interventions are also effective, with favourable cost-effectiveness profiles in the long run. So far, targeted interventions at primary care level have received little attention in Lithuania.

Public health interventions need to become more effective and better embedded

In general, evidence that highly effective public health interventions are actively pursued is limited at all levels. Concrete initiatives have been few or remain described in general terms. At the local level, the responsibility for public health mainly lies with municipalities, who are encouraged to set up and run (or contract if they do not have one) Public Health Bureaus (Kalediene et al. 2011). Lithuania currently has 47 such institutions across the 60 municipalities. However, municipalities are for the most part free to choose the activities they implement and decide on their level of effort. No framework is in place to help ensure that local-level stakeholders implement evidence-based interventions or are accountable for progress on results (as opposed to simply implementation).

A programme has nevertheless been set-up to develop joint health promotion efforts between public health bureaus and PHC providers. Since 2015, once a year, PHC providers can order free of charge diagnostic tests for patients (men aged 40 to 55 and women aged 50 to 65 years) with risk factors for CVDs (obesity, smoking, harmful alcohol consumption). The intervention consists in setting up an individual CVD prevention plan, a suggestion to attend a programme of a health promotion lectures at a Public Health Bureau, and a referral to a secondary care specialist if necessary. Around 1500 people were registered in 2015. In 2017, a similar programme is being launched for people at risk of diabetes. Outside these programmes, the Public Health Bureaus decide on their activities quite freely depending on available budget, with most initiatives focussing on alcohol abuse.

Overall, most public health efforts are geared towards small initiatives which are insufficiently evaluated. Most interventions, such as information sessions on harmful alcohol use or benefits of healthy diet at the Public Health Bureaus, are assessed in terms of process indicators, such as a number of participants, and not with regard to outcomes. Project design, including monitoring and evaluation, must focus also on the effectiveness of these actions. This could improve results, which has been below expectation in many programmes, notably those targeting harmful alcohol consumption. The above-described prevention programmes for patients at risk of CVDs included a comparison of health outcomes (mostly self-reported data) before and after the intervention but it has not been evaluated. Evidence on the effectiveness and cost-effectiveness of public health policies could support decision-makers in implementing the most suitable actions, especially to reduce the alarmingly high alcohol-related harm.

Further priority can be given to increased and stable funding for public health services. Lithuania allocates 1.9% (2016) of health spending to preventive services, noticeably below the OECD average, although this number does not include the ambitious intersectoral collaboration, and prevention efforts in primary care. Many development initiatives and research projects are conducted within time-limited EU funded projects. While project based testing and piloting is good to find effective approaches, there is a risk that many good projects will not be sustained without a more robust financing framework for these functions. The Public Health Strengthening Fund, operational since 2016, is founded to finance disease prevention, social advertising campaigns and health research. The funding comes from an ear-marked share of the alcohol tax and can mitigate dependence on EU grants. But its resources are limited. In 2016, 1.3 million euro was allocated to this fund (MoH). The fund is also, just like EU funding, set up to support projects, not institutionalise services.

Finally, on the public health front, it is worth noting that despite relatively low levels of antibiotic consumption, antimicrobial resistance is a concern in Lithuania. The consumption in the community of antibiotics in Lithuania stands at 16.9 DDD per 1 000 inhabitants per day (2016, ESAC-Net), considerably lower than the EU average (21.9). Yet, the levels of antimicrobial resistance (AMR) for most pathogens under surveillance by the European Centre for Disease Control are high (ECDC, 2017). In 2015, Lithuania introduced nation-wide regional AMR management groups in the regional public health centres, to coordinate expert from different sectors (Hygiene Institute), but further efforts to change clinical behaviour, in both PHC and the hospital sector, are needed.

3.2. Efforts to improve quality must be intensified

This section first describes the main features of the existing quality assurance framework and some recent policies which explicitly aim to improve quality, including efforts to collect and use data on quality. Subsequently, data on quality which allows for comparison with OECD countries is analysed. It generally shows that despite some progress, Lithuania still ranges towards the bottom of the OECD distribution for most indicators.

3.2.1. Lithuania has put in place a number of initiatives to support improvements in quality of care

Policies and institutions to improve quality of care are slowly developing.

The State Health Care Accreditation Agency (SHCAA) is the main institution in charge of quality assurance. The SHCAA, subordinated to the MoH, has long been in charge of licensing of health care organisations and most professionals. Public and private health care organisations must comply with certain input-related requirements – regarding facilities, medical devices, staff – as well as process requirements – regarding governance, quality management, medical audit, clinical care protocols, registration of adverse events, collection of patient feedback, and respect for patients' rights. Health care professionals' licencing requires a minimum number of hours of professional training. The SHCAA can inspect facilities either to investigate patients' complaints or to verify that licencing criteria are met.

The SHCAA has recently launched an accreditation programme, but it seems to attract few providers. In March 2016, an accreditation programme was initiated to promote quality improvement, which is voluntary and currently limited to PHC providers. By the end of 2016, only five PHC organisations had applied for accreditation and ten more were in the preparation stage (Ministry of Health, Lithuania, 2016). In January 2017 a financial incentive in the form of a marginally higher capitation for accredited clinics was introduced, although it seems to be inadequate to substantially raise interest, possibly because of the accreditation fee clinics have to pay. By the end of 2017 only 16 institutions were accredited (SHCAA, 2018).

Some clinical guidelines exist but information about their effective use is lacking. The Ministry of Health has issued 123 diagnostic and treatment protocols (in cardiology, oncology, neurology, traumatology and paediatrics). Providers are encouraged to follow them, regardless of the ownership or level and volume of the services provided. If there are no nationally approved protocols, health care providers are required to prepare protocols themselves for the high risk diagnostic and treatment procedures (Ministry of Health, Lithuania, 2016). No mechanisms are in place to monitor compliance or support providers in implementation. To date, patient safety has received very little attention. Overall, Lithuania lacks a system-wide support for continuous health care quality improvement.

Some initiatives put greater emphasis on measuring and – at least for primary care – rewarding quality

Quality is increasingly monitored and Lithuania in 2017 reported data on a range of OECD-HCQI indicators. In 2012, a set of 15 quality indicators for hospitals was adopted, in line with the PATH (Performance Assessment Tool for Quality Improvement in Europe) recommendations. Quantitative indicators include for instance the frequency of Caesarean sections, mortality from myocardial infarction during active treatment, mortality from stroke during active treatment, and the frequency of development of pressure ulcers. Qualitative indicators pertain to patient satisfaction and the presence of some processes (for instance adverse event reporting system). However, the procedure for engaging hospitals in a quality discussion, limited to a yearly discussion of the results between the managers of the facilities and the NHIF, is weak. Hospital remuneration is not tied to quality. For primary care, a set of indicators is used to calculate a performance-based add-on to the capitation (see below). It is worthwhile highlighting though that in 2017 the MOH participated in the OECD HCQI data collection efforts, the results of which are analysed further below.

Information on quality is shared transparently in an effort to support an informed choice for patients. Quality indicators for hospitals are published annually on the website of the SHCAA. For primary care, many quality indicators are calculated to facilitate bench marking by clinics and municipalities. For example, the Hygiene Institute routinely produces avoidable hospitalisation rates for each municipality. For patients, data on individual facilities' performance is readily available on-line, published by the five territorial insurance funds. While this is a very welcome step towards improving transparency, further steps could be taken to contextualise and make this information interpretation-friendly. For example, the five funds provide different level of detail and present the data in different ways on their respective websites.

PHC remuneration is organised to reward performance, through fee for service and a pay-for-performance component. Facilities receive an age and sex-adjusted capitation rate (72.9% of total PHC facilities' revenue in 2016) with an additional per capita amount for rural facilities (7.1% of revenue). PHC providers also receive activity- or output-based payments for a list of specific services (10.7% of revenue). The list of 63 services which render additional payments includes immunisation, monitoring of pregnant women, early diagnosis of tumours, and home visits by nurses. The final element of remuneration is a result-based payment based on a list of performance indicators (9.3% of revenue). In recent years, the share of capitation in total revenue for PHC providers has declined in favour of higher performance payments.

The performance based payment for PHC is well intended and monitored, and some indicators show improvements. Twelve indicators are taken into account to determine the payment. They include to the proportion of registered adults who visits the clinic at least once per year. For children, the same indicator is used plus one for the share of children who received a dental screening. Four indicators monitor cancer screening (breast, cervical, colorectal and prostate cancer screening) and four indicators relate to results achieved for chronic patients: hospitalisations of patients with asthma, diabetes, hypertension and schizophrenia. Given the burden of disease and the still relatively low screening rates (see below), the focus on non-communicable diseases of the pay-for-performance is welcome. Results are monitored by the NHIF, which for instance show that the cervical cancer screening rate for registered patients rose from 23 percent in 2008 to 35% in 2015. Other screening rates are also improving and hospitalisation rates for chronic diseases are decreasing, albeit slowly. There is however large room for improvement, as compared to other countries (see next section). In the absence of an evaluation framework, the impact of the scheme is difficult to ascertain.

A review and revision of the pay-for-performance component would be warranted. The knowledge base on indicators which should be used for adequately remunerating performance suggests a number of good practices (McColl et al., 1998, EXPH 2017). In particular, the performance criteria should point to results which can be directly influenced by the provider and are sensitive to their level of effort, reflect important clinical areas, but also more generally encourage the delivery of appropriate services. In this regard, the indicators used in Lithuania could be improved. For example, a high share of listed adults who visit PHC over one year, which generates a bonus payment, does not necessarily mean the clinic meets those in most need of a consultation. Furthermore, general check-ups for healthy adults are not shown to improve morbidity or mortality. Finally, access in Lithuania is well developed (previous chapter) and in 2016, 92% of PHC clinics reached the highest level of performance on this indicator. Therefore, the usefulness of this indicator in the performance scheme could – at this point – be debated. As another example, the indicators on avoidable hospitalisations which are certainly relevant to monitor the performance of PHC at a high-level, may not be so appropriate at the level of a single (especially small) facility as they are not only impacted by primary care. Additionally, the denominator (number of listed patients diagnosed with a certain chronic disease) can be affected – and potentially manipulated – in response to the performance scheme, calling its robustness in question. For chronic diseases, performance schemes typically use processes indicators to reward clinical excellence (for example, blood pressure checks for patients with hypertension, tests for HgbA1c for diabetic patient) or better intermediate outcomes (for example, cholesterol control in people with diabetes or controlled blood pressure). So, while monitoring and rewarding performance may be appropriate, the current system could be better calibrated.

Additional measures directly support the delivery of more effective services

In recent years, Lithuania has undertaken two interesting initiatives to strengthen specific services which have a strong potential to increase the effectiveness of service delivery and thus quality.

An EU-funded programme supporting the integration of health and social services has been the main initiative to encourage care co-ordination. In Lithuania, efforts to encourage the coordination of care across health providers are essentially limited to requirements made for providers to communicate with one another when patients move across different parts of the system. In 2013 however, the Ministry of Social Security and Labour launched the Integrated Assistance Programme to offer integrated health and social care to the disabled and elderly. In 21 municipalities, 70 mobile teams provide integrated services (nursing and social care) at home, including support to their informal care givers. Funding from the EU will support the expansion to all municipalities but funding is only secured until 2020. The project-based approach can help devise effective solutions to integrate services, but carry a risk that they may not be sustained. Given the increasing population at need for such services, the programME should be carefully evaluated and – if cost-effective – sustainably funded.

The recently introduced functional clustering can strengthen the quality of specific hospital services for which rapid access is needed. In 2013, a new wave of reforms established standardised pathways for patients who suffer from specific conditions for which a fast response is required, namely stroke and some types of myocardial infarction (with elevated ST). Under the "Integrated Health Care and Functional Cluster Systems", depending on severity, patients are directed by emergency services either to the regional hospital or one of the six regional stroke treatment centres or five cardiology centres established by the programme. They receive an initial treatment and can be later transferred to a facility closer to their home. For strokes, the programme has essentially allowed the development of intravenous (IV) thrombolysis or thrombectomy in the country, two types of procedures used to treat and remove blood clots from the body.

Although a more complete evaluation is required, results are encouraging. According to data provided by the Ministry, the rates of IV thrombolysis, a quality indicator monitored in stroke care which remain disappointingly low in many high income countries (Scherf et al, 2016), has increased dramatically in Lithuania. In 2012, 160 intravenous thrombolyses were performed and in 2016, 808. For thrombectomies the number rose from 4 to 276. Since the creation of Percutaneous Coronary Intervention Centres (open 24/7) for the cardiology patients, the time of access to the required intervention has dropped and hospital mortality in patients is decreasing[2]. The Government plans on expanding this clustering system to all people who suffer from a myocardial infarction. These measures, as well as selective contracting based on minimum volume, hold great potential for increasing the quality of inpatient services in Lithuania but it will be critical to demonstrate more rigorously that they lead to improvements in clinical outcomes.

3.2.2. Despite progress, quality of care indicators still place Lithuania among OECD's poor performers

On the positive side, survey data consistently shows that patients in Lithuania are more satisfied with services than a few years ago. However, results on primary and acute care, as well as across the system, as seen through the prism of cancer, confirm that improving quality in the Lithuanian health system will be the main challenge in the years to come.

The satisfaction of the Lithuanian population in the health system is increasing

A number of European surveys suggest that Lithuanians are more satisfied with their health system than in the past. According to Eurobarometer, the population's view on the quality of health care improved dramatically between 2009 and 2013. Between these 2 years, the share of Lithuanians rating the overall quality of health care in the country as good increased from 40 to 65%, the largest increase among European Union countries, although this share is still below the EU average (71%) (European Commission, 2014). The European quality of life survey (Eurofound, 2017) also shows increased trust in the health care system. On a scale from 1 (very poor quality) to 10 (very high quality), the average rating of the quality of health services in Lithuania has increased from 5.1 to 6.3 between 2003 and 2016, the fourth highest increase in the European Union (Figure 3.8). Patient satisfaction is an important quality metric and the progress shown is surely encouraging. Yet, as the rest of the section will show, results on outcomes of care are not progressing as fast and lag at the bottom of the distribution.

Figure 3.8. The rating of health services quality has increased over time in Lithuania

Quality ratings of health services in European countries 2003 and 2016

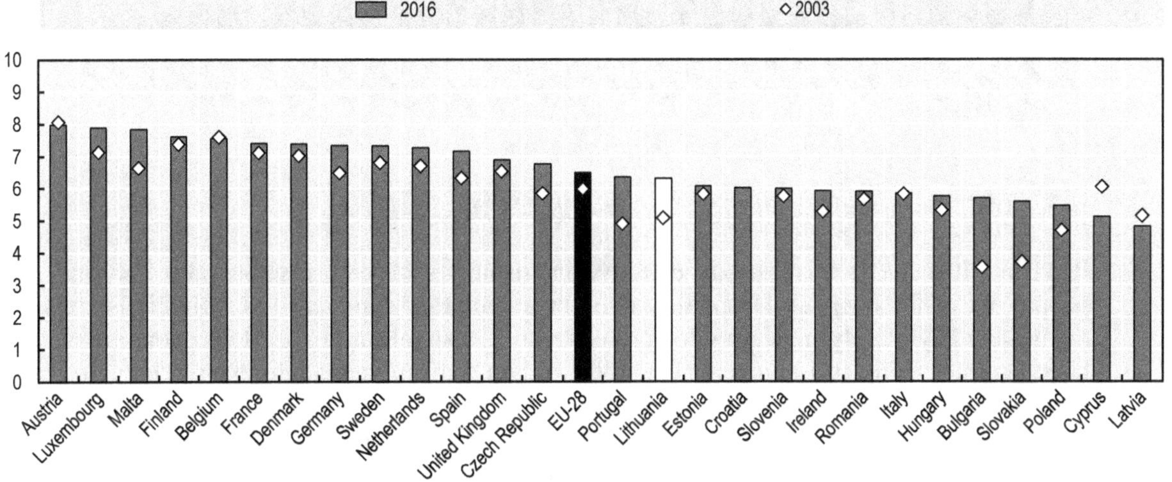

Source: European quality of life survey 2016 (Eurofound, 2017).

Prevention and treatment at the primary care level must still improve

Immunisation rates could be higher. High rates of children immunisation were one of the hallmarks of soviet systems, which many countries have retained. Results in this regard in Lithuania are a bit disappointing and around or slightly below OECD averages: 93 percent of children are immunised against diphtheria, tetanus and pertussis, 94 percent against measles and 94 percent against Hepatitis B – the only rate at par with the OECD average (2015). Although Influenza vaccination coverage for people above 65 is much higher than in Latvia and Estonia, at 19.5% it remains well below the OECD average (Figure 3.9).

Figure 3.9. One of five people over 65 received a flu shot in 2015

Percentage of population aged 65 and over vaccinated for influenza, 2015

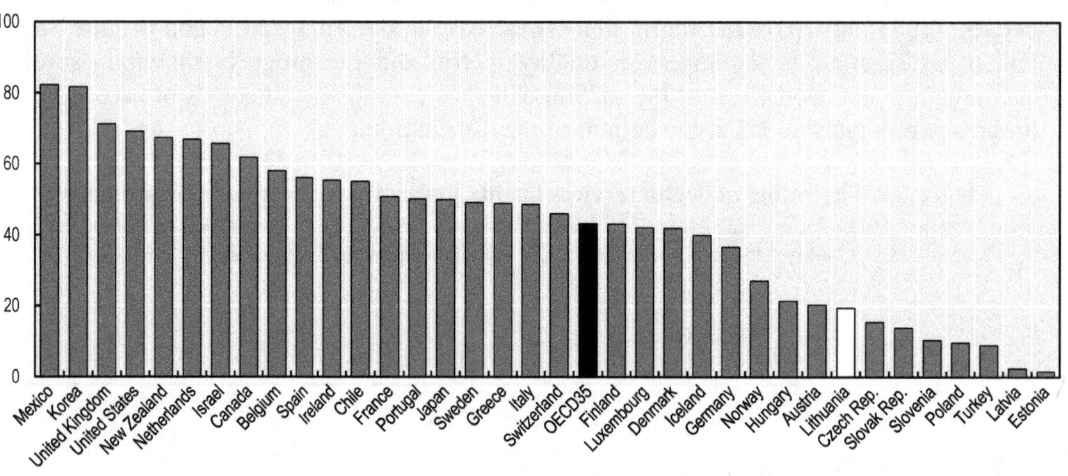

Source: OECD Health Statistics 2017, http://dx.doi.org/10.1787/health-data-en.

PHC in Lithuania is increasingly effective in managing chronic diseases and keeping people out of the hospital. Hospitalisations for ambulatory care sensitive conditions are among the key quality indicators for primary care. Hospitalisations for these conditions have been declining in Lithuania since 2005, although from very high levels. The gains are however unevenly distributed across the country with more modest improvements in rural areas, possibly caused not only by differences in available PHC services but also differences in social conditions and support (Jurevičiūtė and Kalėdienė, 2016).

Lithuanian data submitted to the OECD for the years 2012–2015 confirms that the proportion of patients hospitalised for congestive heart failure, asthma and COPD has been decreasing. For Asthma and COPD, the rates are in fact converging with OECD averages, keeping in mind that this progress is only relative as many countries manage to achieve substantially lower rates of hospitalisations. On the other hand, despite progress, for congestive heart failure, the proportion of patients hospitalised still remains the highest among 32 countries reporting this indicator to the OECD, more than twice the average rate. Hospitalisation rates for diabetes are a third higher than the OECD average and do not seem to decline (Figure 3.10).

Figure 3.10. Hospital admissions for chronic conditions are declining in Lithuania

Age-sex standardised hospitalisation rates per 100 000 population aged 15 and above

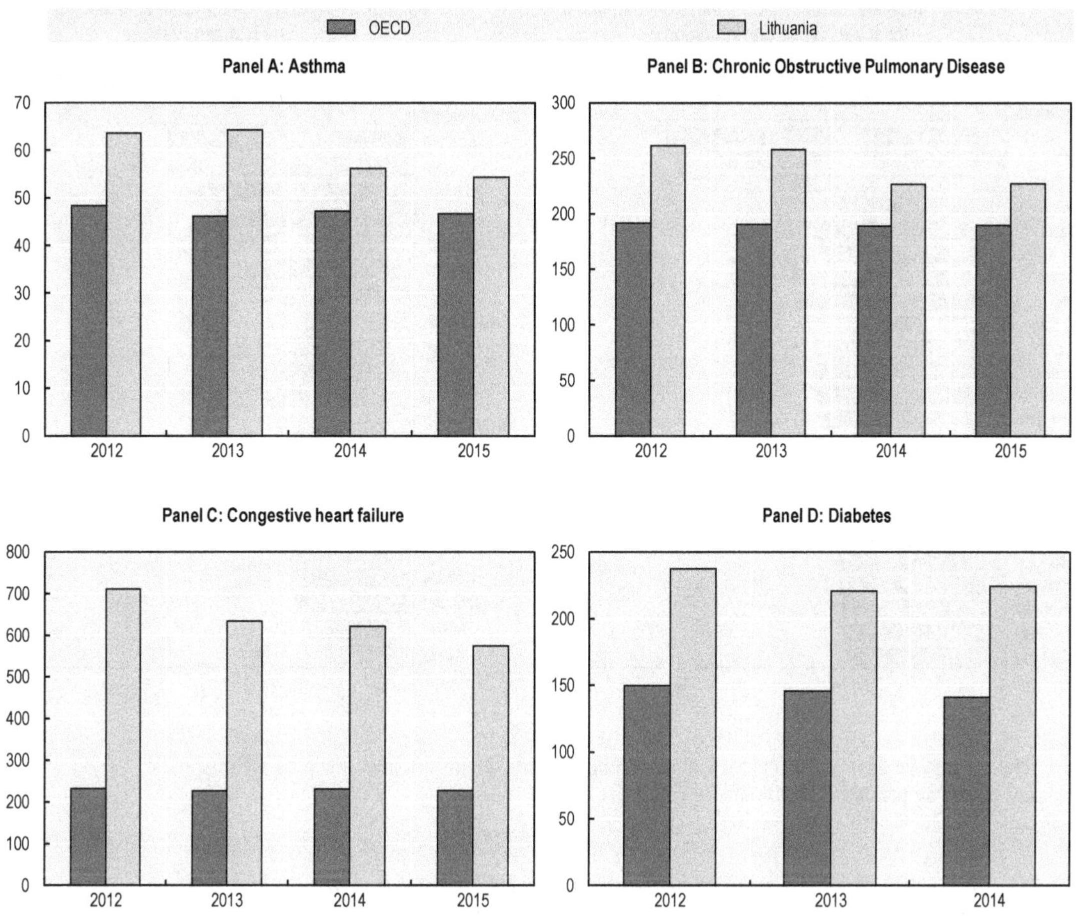

Source: OECD Health Statistics 2017, http://dx.doi.org/10.1787/health-data-en.

Hospital mortality for acute conditions is stubbornly high

The quality of acute health care services also needs to improve. Mortality after hospitalisation for acute conditions is the most common indicator for measuring hospital care quality and is collected by the OECD for international comparison purposes. For the first time, Lithuania provided 30 day mortality data for AMI, haemorrhagic stroke (caused by bleeding) and ischemic stroke (caused by blood clotting) in 2017. In all cases, Lithuania's figures considerably exceed OECD averages. Figure 3.11 for instance shows that Lithuania has the second highest mortality rates of all OECD countries that are able to link mortality data across health providers for AMI and ischaemic stroke. Although Lithuanian data is only available for four years (2012–2015), results have not improved over this period. It will be all the more important to monitor the impact of on-going clustering of stroke and cardiac services. In addition, Lithuania should expand the number of quality indicators reported to the OECD, particularly on patient safety to better benchmark its performance.

Figure 3.11. Thirty-day mortality after admission to hospital for AMI and ischemic stroke are the second highest in the OECD

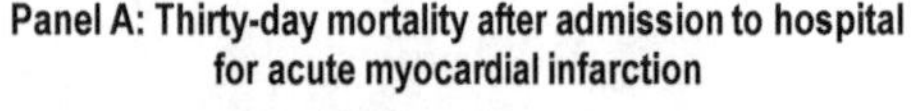

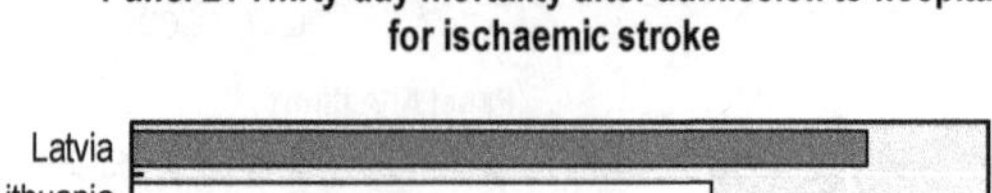

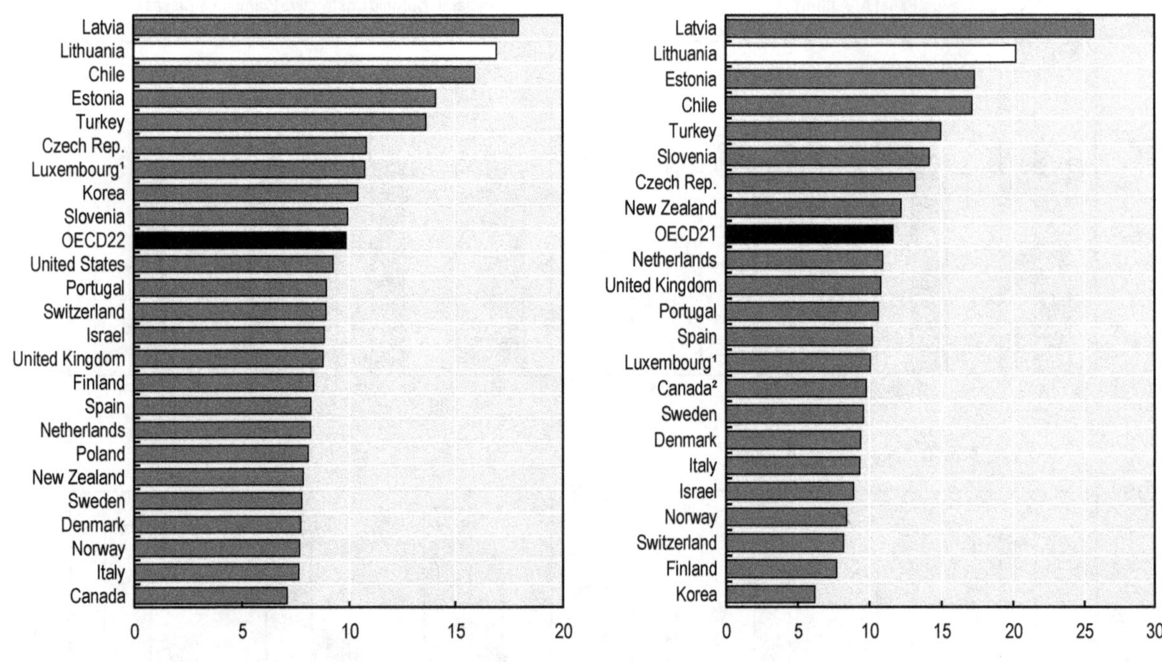

1. Three-year average. 2. Results for Canada do not include deaths outside of acute care hospitals.
Note: Based on patient (linked) data.
Source: OECD Health Statistics 2017, http://dx.doi.org/10.1787/health-data-en.

Cancer care, which relies on both effective PHC and hospital services, is improving although results still lags behind most OECD countries

This section concludes with a disease-oriented perspective on quality by looking at results on cancer care.

Despite progress, PHC providers struggle to ensure better coverage of cancer screening. Lithuania has set up publicly funded population-based screening programmes for common cancers: breast, prostate, colorectal and cervical cancer and coverage of the target population has increased over the last 10 years. In 2015, 45% of targeted women had been screened for breast cancer compared to only 12% in 2006, a significant improvement from very low levels. For cervical cancer, the national screening programme started in 2004 and coverage has increased more slowly, from 43% in 2010 to 48% in 2015. However, these screening rates still lag behind most OECD countries and in both cases, the numbers put Lithuania among OECD's poorest performers (Figure 3.12). According to NHIF data, in 2016, 46% of targeted men were screened for prostate cancer. Colorectal cancer screening, first piloted in 2009 and nation-wide since 2014, is now reaching 43% of the target population.

Figure 3.12. Cancer screening rates for women are low

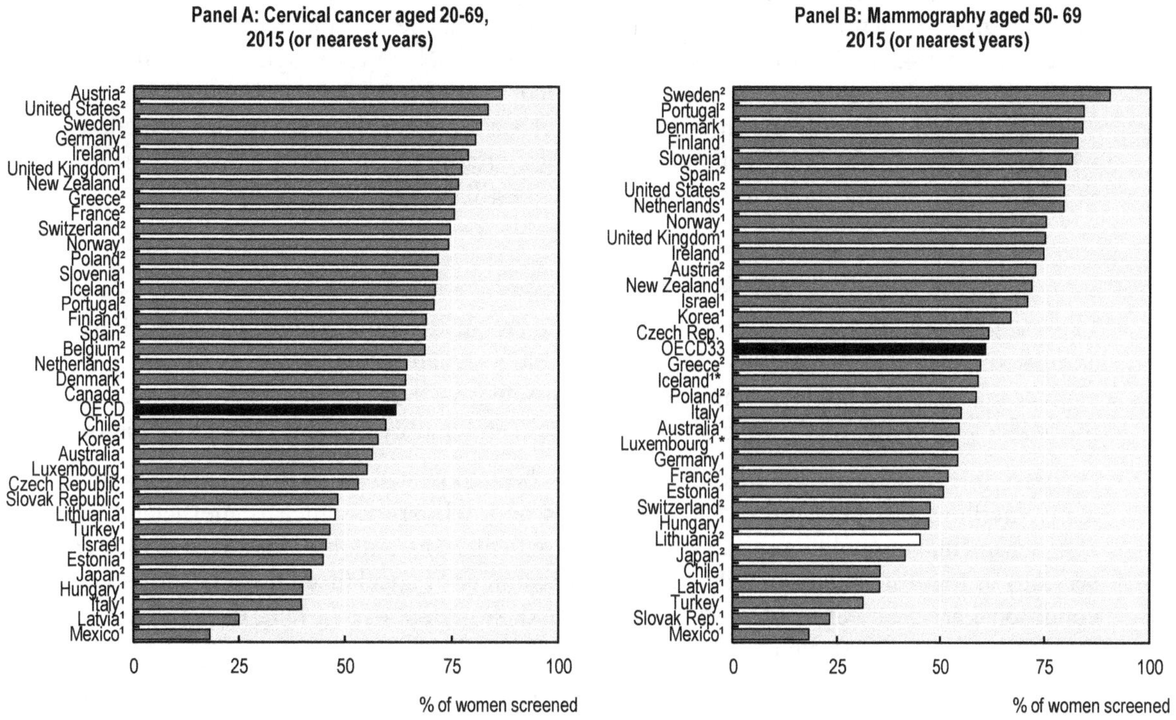

1. Programme data 2. Survey data * Three-year average

Source: OECD Health Statistics 2017, http://dx.doi.org/10.1787/health-data-en.

Primary care is given a large responsibility in the management of the screening programmes but national governance can be tightened to increase coverage and secure equity. Primary care providers have the responsibility to inform patients about the screening programmes and refer eligible patients. They are also incentivised to reach a high uptake through the primary care reimbursement system. All four screening programmes are included in the primary care quality indicators list with a graded payment scale depending on the number of screened people as share of eligible people listed with the clinic. Unlike most other countries with population based programmes, invitations to eligible target groups are not sent through central screening registries, but from the individual primary care centres. Consequently, invitations and follow up for positives are not systematically managed the same way across the country, and take up is to a large extent dependent on the primary care clinic. This also means it is potentially more difficult to automatically link screening data to cancer and other health registries and there is still no screening registry in the country (European Commission, 2017). The National Cancer Prevention and Control Programme (2014–25) is aiming for both improved quality of screening tests and development of the national cancer register, including data linkages to providers and diagnose facilities, among other results. To reach acceptable coverage and equity across the country in this decentralised screening system, more national level steering in addition to the current incentives is probably needed.

Overall, the effectiveness of cancer care quality has improved considerably but still lags behind most OECD countries. Five-year survival rates after cancer diagnosis for most forms of cancer have increased substantially over the past decade and faster than in many other countries, but remain among the lowest in the OECD. Breast cancer survival has increased from 65 to 74% between 2000-04 to 2010-14, but it remains behind those of neighbouring Baltic countries Latvia and Estonia. Similarly colorectal cancer treatment is increasingly successful and at par with neighbouring countries. Colon cancer survival has increased from 45 to 57% in the same time period (CONCORD programme, LSHTM, 2018). For prostate cancer, survival has doubled between the late 1990s and the late 2000s. However, much of the increase in cancer survival is driven by earlier detection, which increases survival also without decreasing mortality (Krilaviciute et al., 2014). All in all thus, from diagnostic to treatment, progress is still needed.

Conclusion

Even accounting for the fact that Lithuania spends relatively little on health, international comparisons suggest that Lithuania should be able to reach better health outcomes. This chapter analyses the policies which aim at improving on the one hand the efficiency of the health system and on the other the effectiveness and quality of the services provided.

Progress in restructuring the hospital sector has been slower than in other countries and many facilities still perform very few surgeries and deliveries, which is inefficient but also detrimental to quality and carries a risk for patients. The ongoing initiatives to cluster services in fewer hospitals, and develop a small number of specialised hospitals for some conditions, are promising but need to be extended, sustained over a long time frame and their actual impact evaluated.

PHC is well organised and reflects best OECD practices with an accessible network of providers and an increasingly team-based approach to care including multiple professions and an extended role for nurses. Several indicators suggest that PHC has a positive impact on wider system efficiency, as shown by the decreasing proportion of patients hospitalised for chronic conditions, such as asthma and congestive heart failure. However, the coverage of preventive services, in particular cancer screening, is still disappointing. Coordination with public health and mental health services has been on the agenda for some time but results are still modest. Actual initiatives to organise coordination tend to be small-scale, seldom evaluated and short-lived. Curbing unhealthy behaviours, such as harmful drinking and smoking, particularly among men, is essential to closing the gap with high performing OECD countries.

The focus on quality needs to be strengthened. A number of initiatives to improve public bench-marking and patient information are implemented in Lithuania but information is not effectively disseminated. The quality assurance culture remains underdeveloped and the policies to change this have not yet been effective. Measuring results and holding stakeholders more explicitly accountable for results can contribute to strengthening clinical outcomes.

Notes

1. Since 2017 cardiology nurses can also work with cardiologists and provide similar services.
2. The question of whether it is decreasing more rapidly than before is not answered.

References

Bunevicius, R. et al. (2014), "Factors affecting the presence of depression, anxiety disorders, and suicidal ideation in patients attending primary health care service in Lithuania", *Scandinavian Journal of Primary Health Care,* Vol. 32, Issue 1.

ECDC (2017), *Antimicrobial Resistance Surveillance in Europe 2015*, Annual Report of the European Antimicrobial Resistance Surveillance Network (EARS-Net).

Eurofound (2017), *European Quality of Life Survey 2016: Quality of life, quality of public services, and quality of society*, Publications Office of the European Union, Luxembourg.

Eurostat (2017), Statistics Explained, Comparative price levels for food, beverages and tobacco, http://ec.europa.eu/eurostat/statistics-explained/index.php/Comparative_price_levels_for_food,_beverages_and_tobacco.

European Commission (2013), "European profile of prevention and promotion of mental health (EuroPoPP-MH)".

European Commission (2014), "Special Eurobarometer 411. Patient Safety and Quality of Care", June 2014.

European Commission (2017), "Cancer Screening in the European Union. Report on the implementation of the Council Recommendation on cancer screening".

EXPH – Expert panel on effective ways of investing in health (2017), Opinion on Tools and Methodologies for Assessing the Performance of Primary Care.

Jurevičiūtė S and Kalėdienė R (2016), "Regional inequalities of avoidable hospitalisation in Lithuania", *Health Policy and Management*, Vol 1, Issue 9.

Jaruseviciene, L. et al. (2014), "Preparedness of Lithuanian general practitioners to provide mental healthcare services: a cross-sectional survey", *International Journal of Mental Health Systems*. Vol 8, Issue 1, No. 11.

Kalediene, R. et al. (2011), "Public health bureaus: new players in health improvement in Lithuania", *Acta Medica Lituanica*, Vol 18, pp183-189.

Krilaviciute, A. et al. (2014), "Cancer survival in Lithuania after the restoration of independence: rapid improvements, but persisting major gaps", *Acta Oncologica*; Vol 53, No 9, pp. 1238-44.

McColl, A. et al. (1998), "Performance indicators for primary care groups: an evidence based approach", *BMJ*; Vol 317.

Murauskiene, L. (forthcoming), Moving towards universal health coverage: new evidence on financial protection in Lithuania, WHO Regional Office for Europe, Copenhagen.

Murauskiene, L. et al. (2013), Lithuania: health system review. Health Systems in Transition, Vol. 15, pp. 1-150.

Medeiros, J and C. Schwierz (2015), Efficiency estimates of health care systems, Economic Papers 549. DOI: 10.2765/49924

National Audit Office (2017), Suicide prevention and aid to individuals related to the risk of suicide, Executive summary of the public audit report (NO. VA-P-10-5-2).

Parliament of the Republic of Lithuania (2016) Decision on the Republic of Lithuania Government's Programme (13/12/2016, No. XIII-82), section 2, Article 31.4, https://www.e-tar.lt/portal/lt/legalAct/ed6be240c12511e6bcd2d69186780352.

Peceliuniene, J. (2011), "Mood, anxiety disorders and suicidal ideation in primary care patients", Doctoral Dissertation, Biomedical Sciences, Medicine. Kaunas, Lithuanian University of Health Sciences.

Rabinovich, L. et al. (2009) The affordability of alcoholic beverages in the European Union. Understanding the link between alcohol affordability, consumption and harms, RAND Europe.

Sassi, F. (ed.) (2015), *Tackling Harmful Alcohol Use: Economics and Public Health Policy*, OECD Publishing, Paris, http://dx.doi.org/10.1787/9789264181069-en.

Scherf, S. et al. (2016), "Increase in national intravenous thrombolysis rates for ischaemic stroke between 2005 and 2012: is bigger better?", *BMC Neurology,* Vol 616, No. 53, http://dx.doi.org/10.1186/s12883-016-0574-7

SHCAA (2018) The State Health Care Accreditation Agency, http://www.vaspvt.gov.lt/node/941 and /882.

ORGANISATION FOR ECONOMIC CO-OPERATION AND DEVELOPMENT

The OECD is a unique forum where governments work together to address the economic, social and environmental challenges of globalisation. The OECD is also at the forefront of efforts to understand and to help governments respond to new developments and concerns, such as corporate governance, the information economy and the challenges of an ageing population. The Organisation provides a setting where governments can compare policy experiences, seek answers to common problems, identify good practice and work to co-ordinate domestic and international policies.

The OECD member countries are: Australia, Austria, Belgium, Canada, Chile, the Czech Republic, Denmark, Estonia, Finland, France, Germany, Greece, Hungary, Iceland, Ireland, Israel, Italy, Japan, Korea, Latvia, Luxembourg, Mexico, the Netherlands, New Zealand, Norway, Poland, Portugal, the Slovak Republic, Slovenia, Spain, Sweden, Switzerland, Turkey, the United Kingdom and the United States. The European Union takes part in the work of the OECD.

OECD Publishing disseminates widely the results of the Organisation's statistics gathering and research on economic, social and environmental issues, as well as the conventions, guidelines and standards agreed by its members.

OECD PUBLISHING, 2, rue André-Pascal, 75775 PARIS CEDEX 16
(81 2018 13 1 P) ISBN 978-92-64-30086-6 – 2018

www.ingramcontent.com/pod-product-compliance
Lightning Source LLC
LaVergne TN
LVHW081412110826
845149LV00010B/1722

* 9 7 8 9 2 6 4 3 0 0 8 6 6 *